AF326526

**To my wonderful children**

# Table of Contents

# DEDICATION

In addition to my children, this text is dedicated to the businessmen/woman that inspired me most;  Mark Cuban, Elon Musk, Peter Thiel, Shanee Moret, & Robert Steve Ivy. Like those I admire, I am committed to enhancing the integrity of the media industry by introducing factually correct information.

Honesty, integrity, and competency will be the hallmark traits of all of my news reporting!

No fake news.  Real Science.  Real Facts!

**Real News!**


David A. Vogel

# ACKNOWLEDGEMENTS

Credit is due to the following experts and other individuals who have provided valuable assistance in putting together this publication. I want to extend each of these individuals a special *"thank you"*:

Q. David Bowers, Richard Chenworth, Steve Contursi, James L Halperin, Robert Steve Ivy, Sam Lukes, Patrick Nielsen, and Scott A. Travers.

A special thank you to my five beautiful children, who serve as a never-ending source of inspiration.

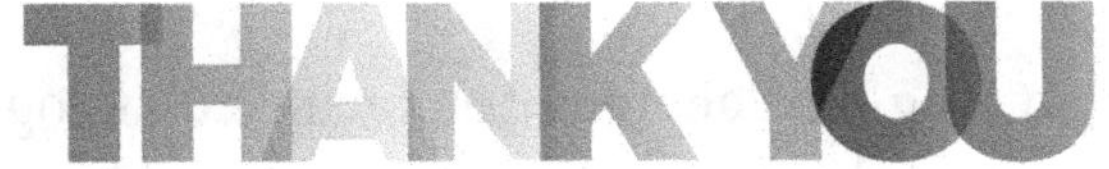

# INTRODUCTION

# CHANGE IS COMING!

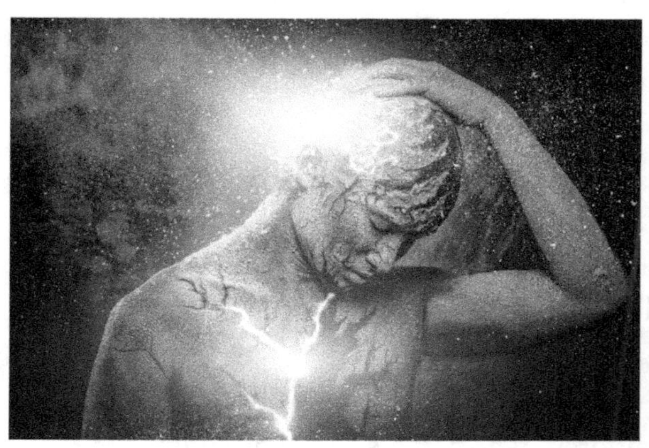

I am the CEO of SharkTV®

Join me in transforming yourself into the ultimate Shark—start acting and thinking like a billionaire.

The coming biotechnology and nanotechnology revolution will bring unprecedented changes to mankind.

Business Sharks, the world's richest men, are

getting ready to defeat this messy business we call "*death*." Learn all about Elon Musk, Mark Cuban, Jeff Bezos, Larry Ellison and the team of scientists working on nanomedical devices and procedures that will repair the human body at a cellular level.

I am going to teach my **Sharks, my loyal fans,** how to live forever. Let's navigate the waters of real science and take the first step to reversing the aging process in your body.

Only **Sharks** will cheat the mortician.

I am going to teach you to be the ultimate **Shark**! The ultimate survivor! You will be rich, healthy, and immortal.

For over 450 million years, there has been one creature on the planet Earth that has survived and adapted to change and lives amongst us today, the **Shark**. A rogue comet might have killed every last dinosaur on Earth, but the **Shark** survived. Since the beginning of time, the **Shark** has been the perfect predator; self-sufficient, always adapting, and always on the hunt...a survivor!!

There are many innovative changes taking place in the world of science and physics. My book will guide you through those changes in simple, easy-to-understand language.

> **Note**: Sign up for my free newsletter, and you will be updated on new events that will impact the way you make important decisions in life. Click below or if you are reading the print version of this book, go to the following URL to get one year of **SharkTalk®** a $289 value absolutely free!
>
> https://sharktv.tv/talk

**You will survive. You will be a Shark!** A **Shark** has a keen sense of awareness. A **Shark** knows that Artificial Intelligence, Biotechnology, and Nanotechnology are becoming so advanced that **Sharks** may very well transcend death by 2045.

Sounds crazy? Not as crazy as you think!! Let me be your guide on this unbelievable journey. You will learn to invest in your own immortality!

But why listen to me?  Why David A. Vogel?

Because I alone have the qualifications to prepare you for this incredible opportunity. I'm an expert in rare collectibles, Cryptocurrency, and economics—my financial acumen has made me a very successful man.

So what? I hear you ask.  There are plenty of successful people in the world.  Sure, but how many have studied physics, quantum physics, astrophysics, and nanotechnology? Not very many is the answer.  Furthermore, my studies in marine biology make me uniquely placed to explain nano-cellular regeneration (spoiler: the ocean holds the secret of eternal youth!). In fact, there's just one person on planet Earth who can weave together the financial and scientific knowledge you'll need to prepare you for the "*Singularity*"...and that's me.

You'll see that I tell it like it is.  Am I blunt? Heck yes!  But that means you can always count on my IMPECCABLE honesty.  I'll give you both sides of the story, and I'll give it to you straight...unlike the news media (and believe me, I'll have more to say about THEM as we go along!).

You see, I believe in the *Fairness Doctrine*. If you know your media history, you might recall that from 1949 until 1987, broadcasters were required to present BOTH sides of a subject. Journalists couldn't just sweep one side of the story under the rug. Our country may have abandoned the *Fairness Doctrine*, but I haven't. I'm here to give you REAL facts, REAL science. If all you're used to is fake news, you better buckle up.

The world is changing quickly, and some of the most exciting breakthroughs are in reversing aging, AI, and similar technologies that will so transform our lives that those who are prepared may live virtually forever. And not only live but live healthily, in young bodies, enjoying a life that people today can only dream of. But you will have to be prepared! My expertise in finance, health, and artificial intelligence make me your perfect guide to prepare for an unprecedented future of health and wealth. You need more than a financial advisor; you need a financial scientist...that is what I bring to the table.  This book will show you how to live rich and live forever.

**Sharks**—This book is for you.

# CHAPTER ONE

# 2045—A PEEK INTO THE FUTURE

**Sharks Will Live Forever**

*"The only thing you can be sure of, so the saying goes,*
*is death and taxes—*
*but don't be too sure about death."*
Joseph Strout, neuroscientist

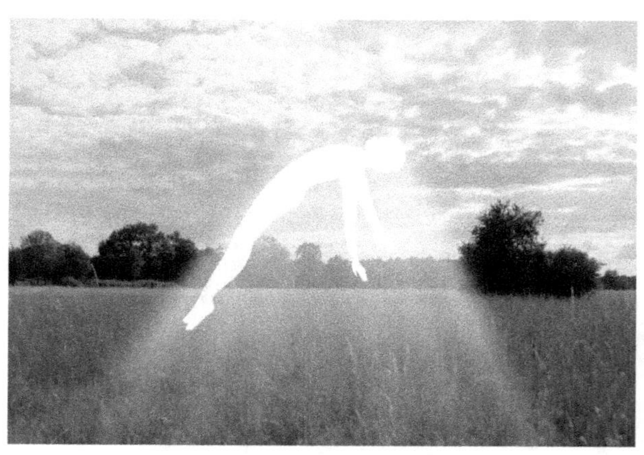

It was a cool New England morning in December. I woke up at 5:00 AM. I was going to have a long day.

Overnight, I had accumulated over 195,200 emails to answer. No problem—my assistant Caitlin, the finest in AI support, reads and responds to all my emails in my personal voice and style. That whole process takes about four minutes. Caitlin then reminds me of my appointments. My personal attendance at any business meeting is optional. That is because Caitlin can create an electronic avatar of me. My virtual self's Artificial Intelligence would pass what is known as the Turing Test. In other words, a panel of experts would not be able to tell the difference between my AI clone and me.

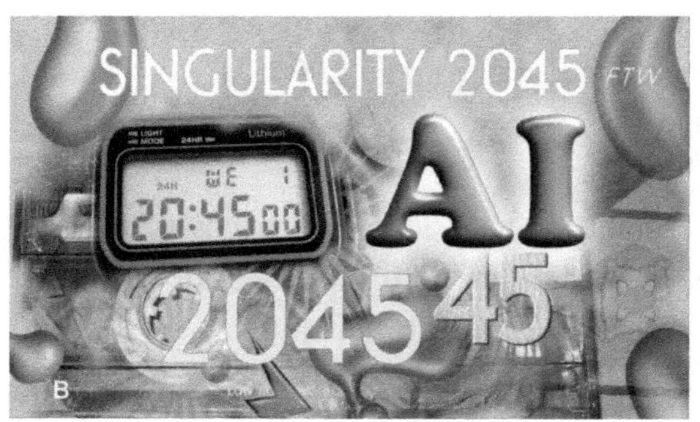


I finally decided against going to my meetings. AI will do it better anyway. Even in 2021 Elon Musk's **GPT 3,** AI can replace the CEO. By 2045, AI is running companies and governments. AI dominates every facet of life.

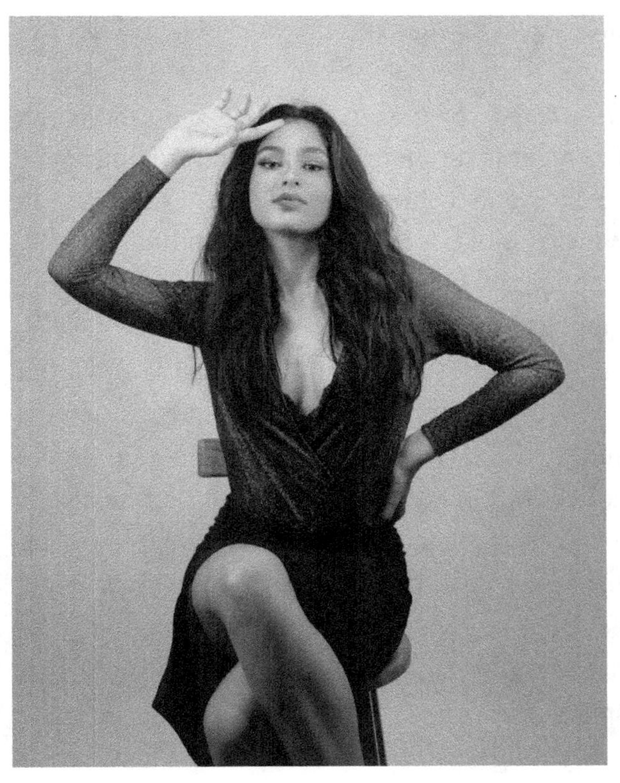

There is one appointment that I am going to keep in person. I am meeting Lucrecia for lunch.

Lucrecia, born in 1945, is a little over 100 years old. When I meet her for lunch, I am graced by a woman of stunning beauty. Her skin and body are that of a very fit and drop-dead gorgeous 23-year-old.   Lucrecia looks like she belongs on the cover of *Sports Illustrated Swimsuit Edition.*   Furthermore, Lucrecia is an incredible brainiac who has nine Ph.D.'s and achieved academic excellence in eleven fields of study, including health, technology, and finance.  Lucrecia speaks five languages fluently, like a native.  She is also very wealthy.  Albeit in 2045, the U.S. Dollar was as ancient as the dinosaur: Lucrecia survived the Great Reset by holding gold, rare collectibles, and virtual *"currency."*  She also is a remarkably talented businessperson—in fact, she is the third-richest woman in the world and is also Elon Musk's second-in-command.  She runs a multi-trillion-dollar-a-week business that spans the globe.  By 2045, AI is running everything on Planet Earth, and Musk is the emperor of AI.

I am obviously attracted to Lucrecia.  She is smart, beautiful, and successful.  Being 15 years her junior in age was hardly relevant. My body frame is mostly well-proportioned muscle.  In fact, Arnold Schwarzenegger, in his prime, never looked as good as I do. Although my technical age was 85, I look like a very fit, very handsome 23-year-old.

Lucrecia and I are part of a rare group of immortals.  In 2040 a secret consortium of the world's richest men and women, led by Elon Musk, made a major breakthrough. Since the beginning of 2000, in one way or another, this group has spent billions of dollars per year perfecting the latest in biotechnology and nanotechnology.  Many great achievements were made along the way.   Cancer was eradicated.  Worldwide famine has ended.  And Green Technology healed our wounded planet. But 2040 was special—2040 was when true nanotechnology became a reality.  And it was a closely guarded secret.

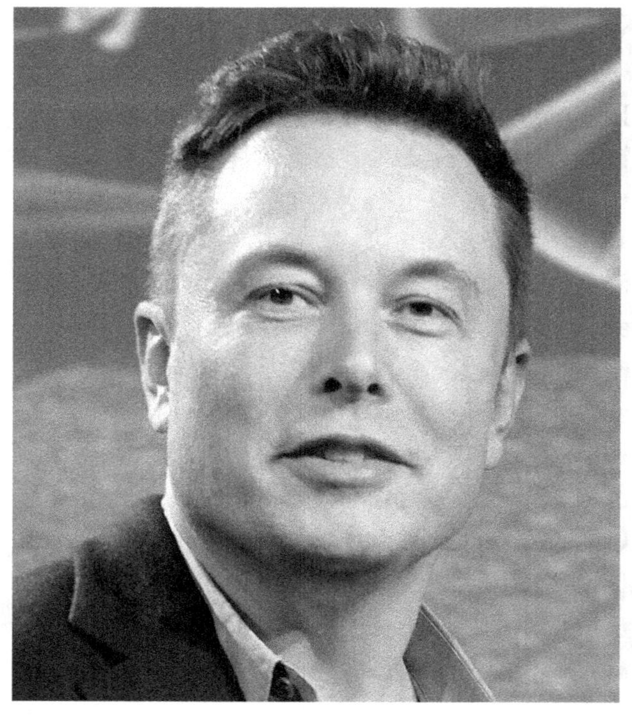

Mastering nanotechnology is mastering control of the very small.  Aging is a disease.  If we can correct the biological problems associated with aging at a nano-level, we can reverse and end that disease.  By mastering control of atoms and cells, Musk and his secret consortium mastered cellular control over the human body and the brain.

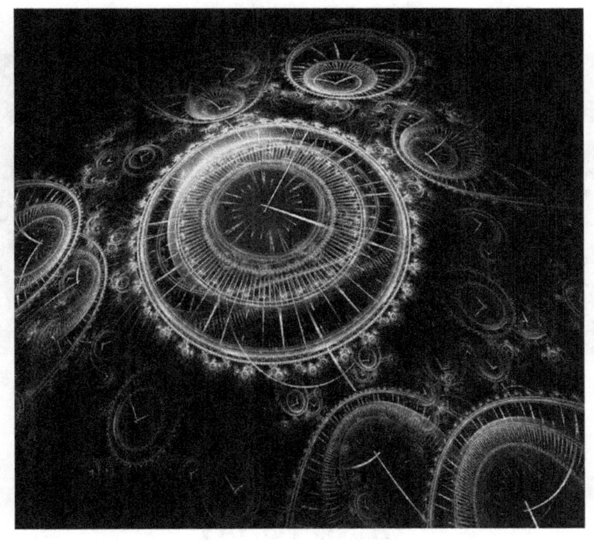

**SHARK TALK: My story is based on the sound science of tomorrow.  The wealthiest people on Earth are investing in nanotechnology.  When we can manipulate cells and particles at the smallest levels, we will control and reverse aging.  This technology is on the horizon and will likely be available in 2045.  Shark's should study biotechnology and nanotechnology.**

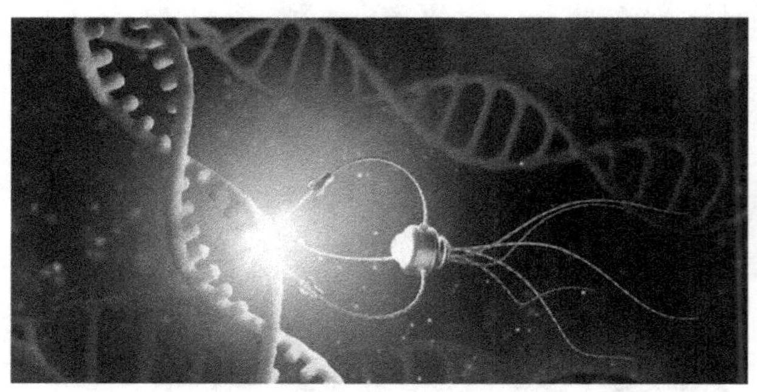

# THE SCIENCE OF TOMORROW IS HERE TODAY

*"I should prefer to an ordinary death, being immersed with a few friends in a cask of Madeira, until that time, then to be recalled to life by the solar warmth of my dear county!*
*But in all probability, we live in a century too little advanced, and too near the infancy of science to see such an art brought in time to its perfection."*
**Benjamin Franklin, in 1773**

Circa 2021, we live in an amazing time.  AI is getting better and better.  Introduced by Elon

Musk, *GPT 3* is the revolutionary AI dominating the market. Elon Musk is changing the way America thinks. Neural links are proven science. It's only a matter of time before man melds with AI. When that happens, man's knowledge will grow exponentially.

Back in 2005, a brilliant scientist and entrepreneur, Ray Kurzweil, predicted that by 2045, humanity would progress to the *"Singularity."* The *"Singularity"* is the ultimate Great Reset. When we reach the *"Singularity,"* man's scientific knowledge will allow him to repair the human body using nanobots, which are robots that are smaller than bacteria in size. Nanobots would rejuvenate your body on a cellular level. DNA transcription errors, one of the leading causes of aging, would be corrected. You would stay a young-looking, healthy person in perpetuity. As long as your body wasn't damaged beyond repair in some sort of freak accident like a piano dropping on your head, you could theoretically live as an immortal.

The science behind Kurzweil's 2045 utopia is sound and realistic—**in fact, the ocean holds the secret to eternal youth**.

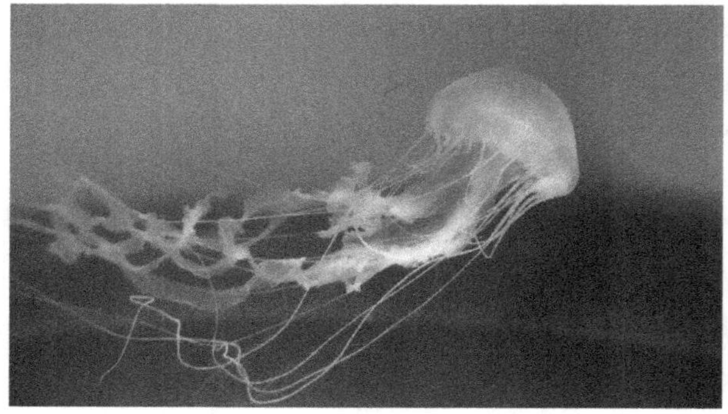

The turritopsis dohrnii (or T-dhornii) jellyfish is an amazing creature. Theoretically, it is immortal. Now, it's not like Superman—if a vicious sea turtle saw a T-dhornii and decided to eat it for lunch, that fish is going to die. But through a process called transdifferentiation, the T-dhornii *"grows young."* It, in essence, reverses the aging process.

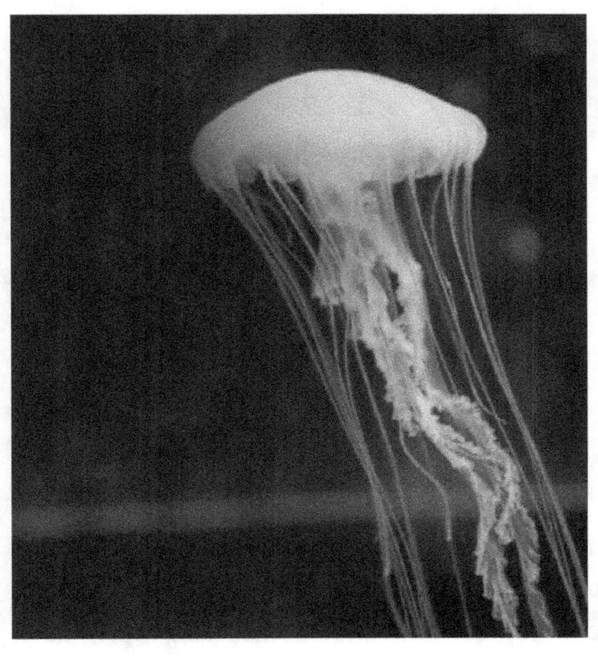

In Ray Kurzweil's 2045, humans have scientifically mastered the ability to transdifferentiate. Ray is not some crackpot. **Bill Gates** called him *"the best person I know at predicting the future of artificial intelligence."* But Gates also called Kurzweil's prediction for a 2045 *"Singularity"* *"optimistic."*

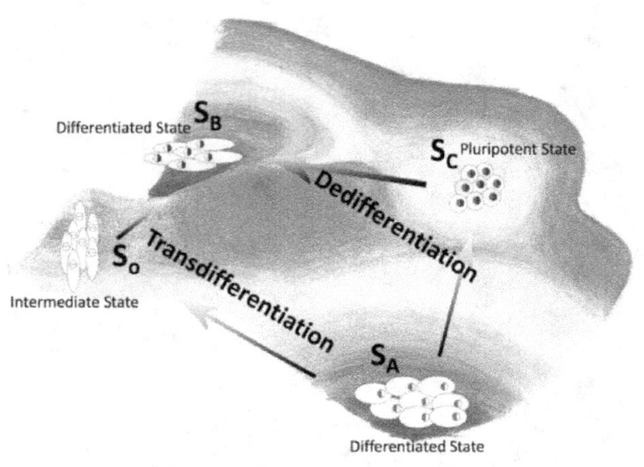


The *"Singularity"* is inevitable. Ray Kurzweil has made predictions before about technological advancements and has been correct. Many of the technological marvels Kurzweil predicted to occur today are quite real. However, much of the technology Kurzweil felt would be ubiquitous in 2021 is only available to the elite and connected. What is *"optimistic"* about Ray Kurzweil's 2045 *"Singularity"* prediction is that he naively believes that scientists will make this life-changing, cutting-edge technology available to the masses and that the inevitability of death will be eradicated for most of the population.

My viewpoint is that Ray Kurzweil will be 100% right about one thing. In 2045, the ability to transcend aging will be a scientific reality. But I do not see this marvelous technology being ubiquitous. As opposed to being available to everyone at virtually no cost, "*immortality*" will be **extremely expensive**. And social acceptance by the elite group that controls immortality technology will be paramount if you are going to survive. Billionaires who can afford the price tag but are disliked or politically inappropriate will be shunned and blackballed.

**SHARK TALK: Plan on being very wealthy if you are going to participate in the "*Singularity*." And make lots of friends—very influential friends. Start today! A Shark will plan for the "*Singularity*" by formulating a sound financial plan. A Shark is also going to seek out other Sharks for friendship. Remember that obtaining wealth is only one element. You must make the right friends.**

**Back to 2045 and my lunch with Lucrecia ..
.**


My date was lovely and delightful.

Lucrecia was 60 years old in 2005 when she first heard about the *"Singularity."* She and I were a lot alike. We believed the technology of the future would extend life for a millennium, but we both had to make it to the point where that technology will be available. That meant staying in perfect health.

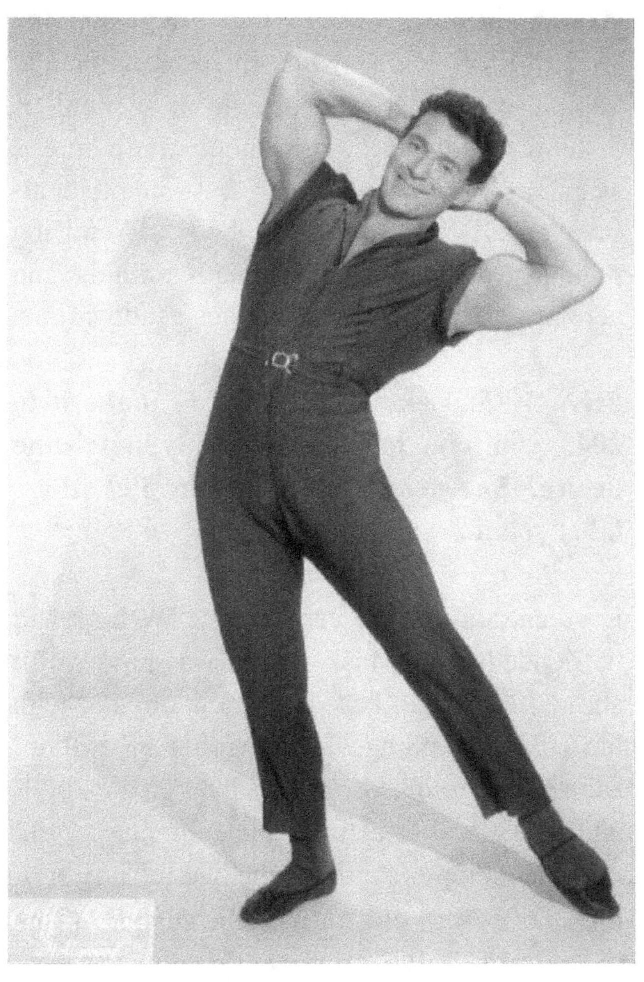

Back in the early 2000s, Lucrecia and I learned everything we could about health and fitness.

And for decades, we were both fanatics about staying healthy.  The first bridge to the "*Singularity*" is staying in perfect health. Taking care of your body in a meticulous fashion.  Being fastidious about what you eat. Managing micro-nutrients and supplements scientifically.  Cleansing the body. Exercising regularly.  Doing both strength training and aerobics and keeping your organs healthy.

**SHARK TALK: If you want to make it to 2045, you have to keep your body in pristine health.  You need to be a fanatic.  Let others label you a "health nut."**

Lucrecia and I were very lucky.  We both had befriended Elon Musk.  Elon was now worth about $20 trillion based on 2021 dollars, with his Bitcoin holding alone topping $3 trillion. Elon spent billions of dollars back in the 2020s and 2030s perfecting biotechnology and nanotechnology.  And now he had the power of life and death.  But in the real version of the "*Singularity,*" Ray Kurzweil's utopia is not reality.  Only the rich and very lucky get to live like a "***God.***"

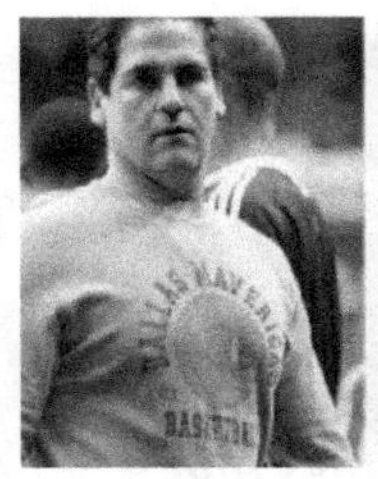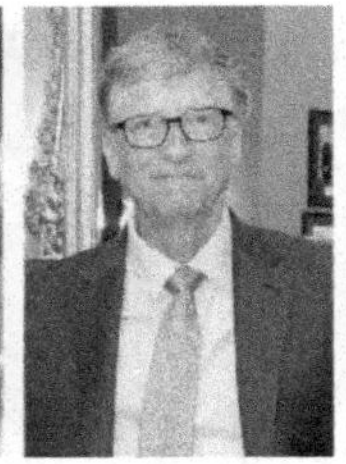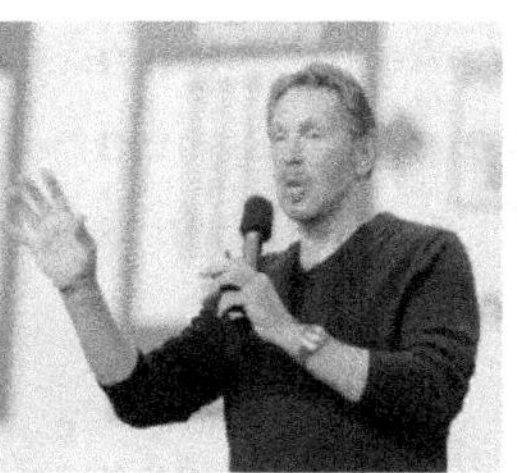

Mark Cuban, Bill Gates, and Larry Ellison all bought their way into the immorality club. Donald Trump offered the equivalent of five billion 2021 dollars to get an invitation, but no one wanted him to be part of this elite group. Donald had angered the wrong people and had too many powerful enemies. Being rich wasn't enough.  You had to have a  friend, someone connected, who would sponsor you.

Lucky, a lot of billionaires and trillionaires have been reading my books and were fans of my hit Podcast **Shark TV®**. Many of my die-hard fans took a liking to me. It pays to be a celebrity author and consultant. I met the right people. Elon Musk became one of my greatest fans.

SHARK TALK:  **If you want to be able to avail yourself of 2045 technology, you will have to know the right people. The time to**

make new friends is now.  Reach out.  Make
yourself known.  Be a Shark.  Remember:
Sharks like to be friends with other Sharks.



*"It is one of the most remarkable things that in all
of the biological sciences, there is
no clue as to the necessity of death."*
**Richard Feynman**

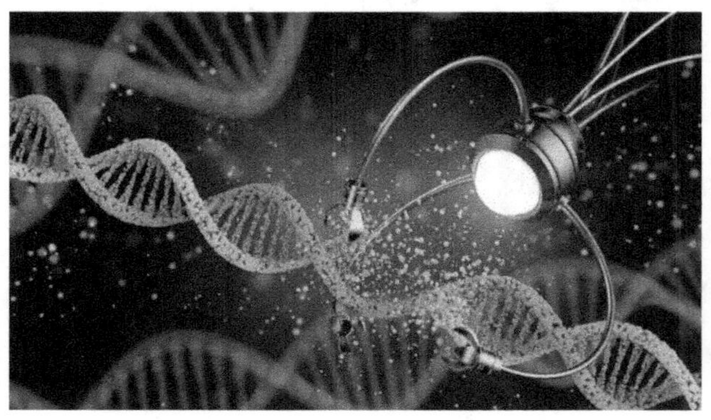

Lucrecia was very special to me.  She
introduced me to Elon Musk personally.  She
made sure I was chosen for *"the procedure."*

*"Lucrecia,"* I said.  Let me tell you why I
wanted to meet you. *"Donald Trump, he wants
in."*

*"David, are you kidding me?   Mark (Cuban) would never allow it."*

*"Lucrecia, please, let's make this simple. Donald wants Mark to have his flagship Trump Tower Apartment and, in fact, Mark could have the whole building!"*

*"Stop it ...let's talk about something else,"* Lucrecia replied.

*"Lucrecia, please get this done.   It is not personal; it is business.   We need Donald's silence.   Imagine what would happen if what we are, what we can do, ever got out?"*

*"OK, David, say no more; I will get it done."*

It was important to keep nanotechnology a secret.  If word got out that only the rich and connected would live forever and everyone else would eventually die, there would be chaos in the streets, riots in every major city, and looting would break out everywhere.   Humanity's transcendence into immortality, for the sake of world order, could never be made common knowledge.

Lucrecia and I reminisced over the events of the past few decades. Notable memories we discussed included:

**<u>June 2021</u>**: I launch my book *Thriving During The Great Reset.* Little did I know that the richest people on planet Earth would read this bestseller. I predicted the U.S. Dollar will be Reset to zero within 10 to 20 years, maybe less. I also launched **Shark TV®** that same year and became an instant celebrity. **Shark TV®** teaches the public to be financial **Sharks**.

**<u>April 2031</u>:** The U.S. Dollar loses all its value ten years after I made this prediction in 2021. The U.S. and World Economy from 2021 to 2031 becomes exponentially worse every year. Finally, the U.S. Government Declares Emergency Action—the U.S. Treasury announces it has Reset the United States Dollar. Federal Reserve Notes are no longer legal tender. Any money you have in the bank has been Reset to zero. The U.S. Government cannot pay its debts. Treasury notes are declared worthless. Social Security and Medicare are no longer able to function. Martial Law is declared.

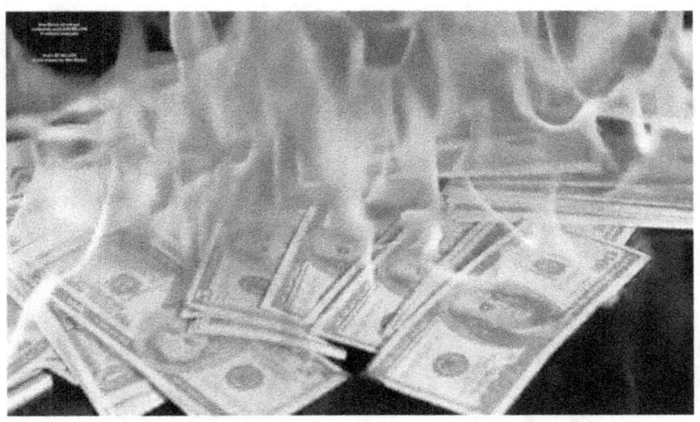

Bitcoin is now trading at what would have been one million U.S. dollars before the Reset. Gold is the equivalent of $50,000 per ounce in 2031. People do not trust government currency, even in its virtual form. Celebrity coins are very popular. Number one on the list is the Elon Musk coin worth about 600,000 of our current dollars. Of course, this author's Bitclout celebrity coin is trading at a close second. Hint: be a big spender and have some fun. **Buy David A. Vogel coin when it is issued.** **Remember**: IN VOGEL WE TRUST®

**June 2033**: Neural Link becomes ubiquitous. In 2021 Elon Musk announced Neural Link. Years earlier, students at the Massachusetts Institute of Technology's lab demonstrated how a computer could translate thoughts in the brain to written text. Both methods were crude, but by 2033, the link between man and machine would make *Star Trek* fans drool.

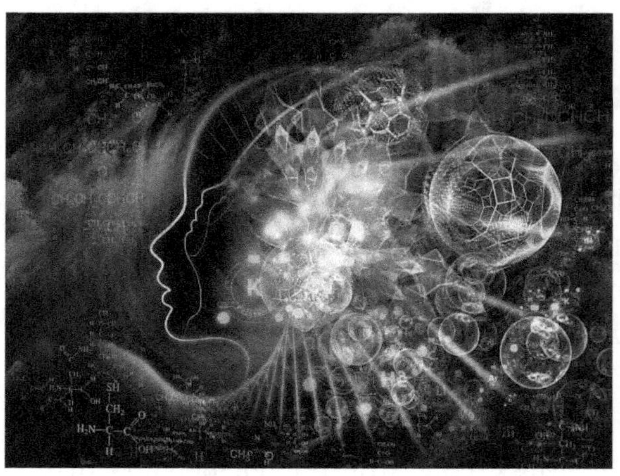

AI can now basically read your mind. You can never lie. All the facts and events you witness are stored in the brain's neurons, which AI can read like an open book. You will have no privacy if the government decides to probe your brain. But only wrong thinking is punished. As part of liberal criminal reform packages, prisons are eventually eliminated. Instead, people who do not conform are sentenced to a virtual reality of hard labor and reconditioning. They are put on the shelf and discarded. In 2033 laws are enacted that dictate how the population should think. You can no longer think for yourself. There are certain norms, and you are expected to conform. Violent crime virtually ended in 2033. Criminals who commit violence can't escape brain probes. Jim Halperin's "*The Truth Machine*" becomes a reality.

AI Neural Links can also be very rewarding and pleasurable. In 2033, Neural Link will offer full-immersion virtual reality. Neural Link would create signals to the brain as if you were experiencing reality. You would see, feel, smell, and taste everything you came in contact with virtually. If you wanted to have a romantic evening with Shakira or Kate Upton, a computer could provide a simulation that would be indistinguishable from reality. People end up getting addicted to VR.

**January 2034:** Biotechnology Takes a Quantum Leap. Cancer is cured. In fact, most diseases are cured. Microbots (which are much larger than the future nanobots) clean the heart and repair it. Growing organs is easy. Aging can be slowed down, but not yet reversed. By 2034 organic gene manipulation will be perfected. Curing disease at a cellular level through somatic gene therapy, cloning, and CRISPR technology, the average human lifespan has Reset to 234 years for those who can avail themselves of the latest in medicine. Unfortunately, most of the world will never

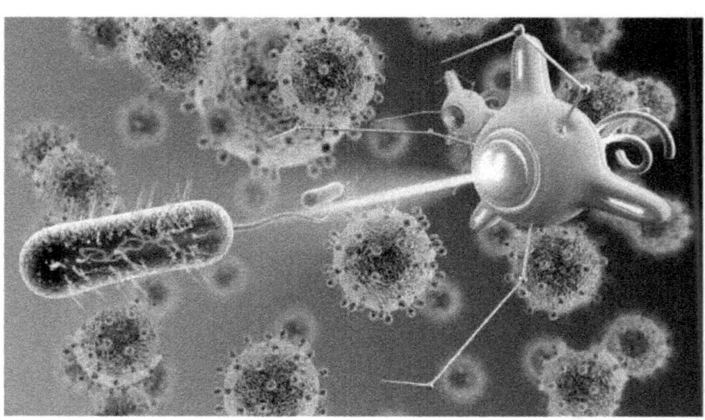

know of this marvelous technology. Those who participate in biotechnology advances cross the second *"bridge"* to the *"Singularity."*

**February 2040:** The final *"bridge"* to the *"Singularity,"* mastering nanotechnology, becomes the greatest breakthrough in science man has ever experienced. Man and machine meld. Man theoretically can become immortal because he can now transdifferentiate. Scientific advances make **"Gods"** out of men.

**October 2045:** Since the U.S. Dollar lost all of its value in 2031, most entrepreneurs deal in Cryptocurrency. Of course, Bitcoin is very prevalent, and one of the few forms of *"currency"* still around that maintained its value. In 2045, a single Bitcoin traded for $5.3 million (based on the value of the new "reset" dollar). Elon Musk's Bitclout coin traded for $6 million per coin. For those of you who trusted in VOGEL, my creator coin is now trading at $4.6 million each. Those of you who bought my book in 2021 and gambled a small amount on my celebrity coin have developed great wealth from a meager investment. Most of my readers, as a *"tip"* to me, put a few hundred to a few thousand dollars into VOGEL coin. Every $100 investment is now worth tens of millions of dollars.

Lucrecia and I shared dinner and memories. We talked about the day's news. Elon Musk's next big project was breaking the speed of light.    Naturally, if humanity is going to radically extend its lifespan, eventually we are going to have to populate other planets. Elon had that all covered.   Warp drive was on the horizon.

*"If I were setting out today to make that drive to the West Coast to start a new business, I would be looking at biotechnology and nanotechnology."*
**Jeff Bezos**

# CHAPTER TWO

# RADICAL LIFE EXTENSION

*"Death is a great tragedy…a profound loss…
I don't accept it…I think people are kidding
themselves when they say they are comfortable
with death."*
**Ray Kurzweil**

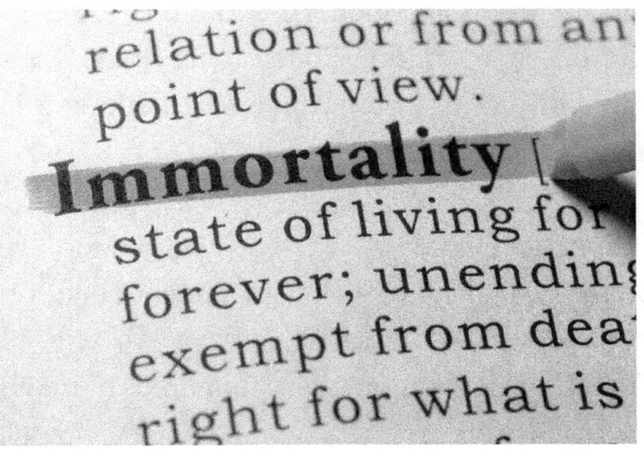


The purpose of my book is to teach you to be a
**Shark**.  A **Shark** wants to live forever.

Of course, theologically speaking, if you believe in Divine Intervention, you also believe man is destined to be immortal. **But part of that destiny may be achieved through scientific advancement**. The concepts of a Creator and Science are not contradictory. In fact, if you studied particle physics and astrophysics as I have, you would realize that the Biblical account of Genesis, for example, describes what scientists call *"the big bang."* To expand and explain what I mean in detail would be the subject of another book. I will end up discussing Genesis and the Big Bang in one of my upcoming Podcasts on **SharkTV®**. **The subject is fascinating, and I know a lot about this topic.**

I do believe God's Great Reset ultimately will be the best reset of all. I am a devout believer, but I do not necessarily believe we will see Divine Intervention for hundreds, maybe thousands of years. It could be longer; it could be sooner. No one knows for sure.

One thing I do know for sure is that for thousands of years, the faithful have predicted that God's Great Reset was imminent. In the year 500 Hippolytus of Rome preached that the Second Coming was arriving that very year based on an analysis of Noah's Ark. Moving forward, in the year 1000, there was another call by religious leaders who were sure that year marked a transition into a new world. After 1001, the embarrassed clerics apologized for their "*mistake*." The new date for God's Reset was set for 1033—exactly one thousand years after the death of Jesus Christ. History shows us that 1033 passed without incident.

For the next several hundred years, preachers would tout that the "*end times*" were just around the corner. No one created the massive following as William Miller did in the early 1800s when he predicted the exact date of God's Great Reset—October 22, 1844. During that early part of American History, much of the population was very religious and very naive. Fake News was easy to spread, and people would not question the word of their preacher. At the time of Miller's sermons, meteorites would shower the Earth, providing a visual spectacle that looked like a "*sign from God*." Millions of faithful followers were awe-struck.

When October 22, 1844, passed, many "*Millerites*" developed depression and anxiety. American media called the passing "*The Great Disappointment.*" Most of the original "*Millerites*" split up into two groups. One is what is known today as the *Seventh Day Adventist Church.* The second group was created by Pastor Charles Taze Russell, who seized the opportunity to lead a large portion of the "*Millerites.*" Russell boldly claimed a firm date for God's Great Reset in 1874, which once again never happened.

The "*Russellites*" eventually became what is known today as the *Jehovah's Witnesses.* Representatives of *Jehovah's Witnesses* first claimed that 1914 was the year of God's Great Reset. Later, during my youth, this very same group "*clarified*" their position, claiming that God's Great Reset would be witnessed by individuals who were alive in 1914. These days, since very few living individuals were born on or before 1914, this group is now arguing "*generations overlap.*" In other words, they gave themselves another extension.

# SCIENCE IS A GIFT FROM OUR CREATOR



*"The more I study science, the more
I believe in God."*
**Albert Einstein**

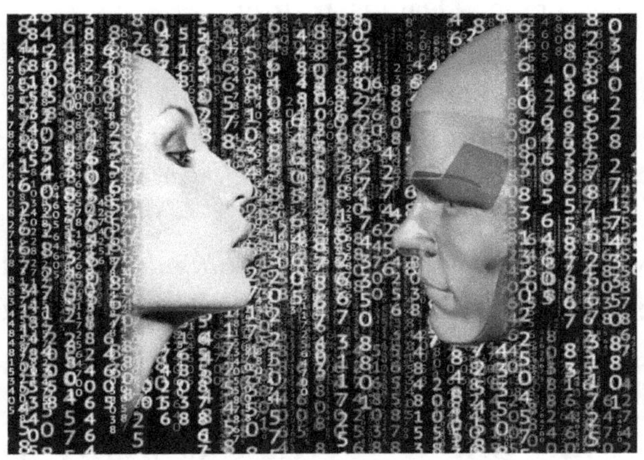

I am opposed to anyone that thinks science is anything but a beautiful act of **Divine Intervention**. Frankly, I am not satisfied with my fragile body, which will operate less efficiently over time. I don't want to move slower, lose mental agility, and experience a loss of sensory acuity. I want to run fast, build my body like a champion, and have sexual desires in perpetuity. Likewise, I want my mind to be sharp, my hearing to be clear, and my vision to be sharp. I refuse to embrace aging as a naturally beautiful life event.

To quote the lyrics of a Rolling Stones hit song, "*What a Drag it is Getting Old.*" Aging is catastrophic. Death is a "*drag.*"

**"*We have the technology. We will make him better than he was before. Better, Stronger, Faster*"**
**Opener for the *Six Million Dollar Man***

Man's Great Reset and the "*Singularity*" will occur long before God's Great Reset. Aging is a disease, and science will be able to cure it.

**SHARK TALK: I refuse to believe an intelligent Creator intended the gift of transdifferentiation to benefit a fish. Altering bad DNA or genes will save lives and rejuvenate the body. In time, you will be able to transdifferentiate. Follow this simple plan if you want to live forever; 1. Educate yourself—keep abreast of the latest scientific innovations. Read Shark Talk®, my insider's newsletter. 2. Get wealthy—it is going to be astronomically expensive. 3. Make lots of friends—you are simply not**

going to be included unless you are well-liked by the powers that control science. Start associating with more talented, intellectual, and successful people.

*"You know things are going to be different!....
No, No, I mean really different!*
Mark Miller, Scientist to Eric Drexler,
Nanotechnology Researcher

*"The net effect of these nanomedical interventions will be the continuing arrest of all biological aging, along with the reduction of current biological age to whatever new biological age is deemed desirable to the patient, severing forever the link between calendar time and biological health. You may still eventually die of accidental causes, but you will live at least ten times longer than you do now."*
Robert A. Freitas, Jr.
Nanotechnology Theorist at University of California

*"The height of stupidity is most clearly demonstrated by the individual who ridicule something he knows nothing about."*
Albert Einstein

## IT'S ELON'S WORLD;

# WE ARE ALL JUST LIVING IN IT

The global skincare market is expected to hit more than $183 billion by 2025.  Each year, human beings flock to their local pharmacies, grocery stores, spas, and salons hunting for the best beauty and anti-aging products the market can offer.  Why is this?  It is because human beings are psychologically wired (read: borderline obsessed) with combating natural aging processes.  We want to look and feel young and beautiful and hide from all those nasty reminders that we will shrivel up and die one day.

Our fear of death is pervasive; it is why Spanish explorer Juan Ponce de León went looking for the *Fountain of Youth*.  It is the same reason why aging celebrities replace their body parts every few years, and it is why the skin cream market is going to hit a quarter billion dollars in our lifetime.  People want to look young forever, even if they cannot stay young forever.

Until recently, most individuals—the scientific community included—have resorted to trying to *mask* the effects of aging rather than do anything substantial to slow them down or stop them altogether, literally.  This makes sense, as it is science fiction to think there is a way to stop one of the most natural processes in the universe: the Circle of Life.

Right…?

Wrong.  We are officially approaching *Altered Carbon* territory.  Now, scientists, with the backing of extremely wealthy individuals who do not want to die (maybe ever), have devised new methods to slow, stop, and yes, even reverse the aging process altogether.  Really.

Now, some of you are still probably thinking, *"this sounds insane."* Our whole lives, we have been told that Father Time is undefeated, and now people are here saying he is about to go down for the count? What gives?  You may be asking, *"what type of occultist psycho-babble are you spewing?"*  When people talk about *"playing God,"* this is what they must mean.

How is this all possible, you might be wondering? Well, as you will read more about below, most of the approaches being explored work on a cellular level and involve our actual genes themselves being targeted by one therapy or another.  Think of it like this—imagine you are a car.  You can periodically change the oil, belts, chains, and spark plugs to extend the vehicle's life for hundreds of thousands of miles, but at some point, the engine will give out, and that is going to be that.  Keeping up with those superficial pieces of maintenance is about as much of a financial commitment as many are willing to make regarding their vehicle.  Changing much else is too expensive, and the older the car becomes, the less cost-efficient it is to fix.  But what would happen if you did start to change those other parts?  What if you changed the engine itself as it started to deteriorate?

Moreover, what if you could manipulate the very atoms and molecules that comprised the car to ensure they never deteriorated in the first place?  Wouldn't that be even better?  What if you could fill the car with gasoline that cleans the tank and use oil that not only prevents metallic friction but restores the worn-out components?  Are you starting to get the picture?

Imagine a car that drove forever, never succumbing to the salt on the roads, gunk in the engine, or rust on the metal. This is what modern biologists and molecular scientists imply we, as human beings, can do with our bodies. Some are saying we can cruise the highway of life forever.

The technologies we are going to talk about are a little heavy. This science is cutting edge, and the big ideas being promulgated are stacked with terms that might sound like something being studied in places like Area 51. However, we can assure you that the individuals working to combat the effects of aging discussed here deal with real, actual science. **Science fiction is becoming a science fact right before our eyes.**

Some of the most brilliant people in the world, with the backing of some of the wealthiest people in the universe, are already working on this, and they have been at it for years. Billionaire Amazon CEO Jeff Bezos and PayPal co-founder Peter Thiel are among the wealthy elite that has invested in this research, so you can bet your bottom dollar that this is serious business. These guys do not mess around, and if they are on board, you better believe that the science is credible, vetted, and promising. You do not become a billionaire investor by throwing money at pseudo-science. You do it by backing the right horses and reaping the benefits once those horses cross the finish line.

According to an article from CNBC, Bezos and Thiel are mutually backing a San Francisco-based company called *Unity Biotechnology*, which is working to, quite literally, *"extend human healthspan, the period in one's life unburdened by the disease of aging."* They want to kill dying. Unbelievable.

Famously, Thiel once convened a summit of 12 *"eclectic"* scientists engaged in research that some might describe as *"radical."* In contrast, some others might even call it *"heretical"* to attempt to devise ways to defeat the effects of aging. It was a meeting of the minds unlike any that has ever taken place in the history of humanity.

*"Among the guests was Cynthia Kenyon, a molecular biologist, and biogerontologist who had garnered attention for doubling the life span of a roundworm by disabling a single gene. Aubrey de Grey, a British computer scientist turned theoretician who prophesied that medical advances would stop aging. And Larry Page, co-founder of an internet-search darling called Google that had big ideas to improve health through the terabytes of data it was collecting,"* reads a retelling of the events in news magazine *The Week*.

The research began to proliferate. What was happening around the world was revolutionary, and it was starting to catch on. Another company cited in that same CNBC report, Calico, has taken in *"hundreds of millions"* of dollars supporting anti-aging research from the co-founder of Oracle, Larry Ellison. Again, investments of that magnitude are examples of an authentic, genuine commitment to this science. The difference between theoretical pipe dreams and real, actual progress is, quite bluntly, money.

All of this adds up to many powerful people looking to do some amazing things. So far, the results are extremely promising. Below, we will look a little closer at how scientists hope to accomplish these future medical marvels. What you will find is that they are going to do it with some …

## BIG IDEAS AND VERY, VERY SMALL SOLUTIONS

It should not be surprising that the pillars of anti-aging (and reversing aging) research are formed in the smallest parts of the human body. Researchers are working to manipulate the building blocks of human life on a molecular level and restructure, reform, and repair our cells.

The two primary areas of research being explored are biotechnological and nanotechnological. In simple terms, one relates to manipulating our cells, genes, and biological matter on a fundamental level, and the other deals more with sending incredibly small nanobots into our bodies to augment, improve and protect our natural functions.

Research into the biotech sector involves re-growing cells and tissues, sometimes replacing them with the same technology used to clone larger pieces of organic matter. In other instances, the aim is to shut off specific genes by manipulating their messenger ribonucleic acid (mRNA). Turning off genes sounds like a bad thing, but it is one of the most promising research areas with respect to anti-aging.

In that same vein, a research paper by Dr. Michael West, CEO of BioTime, Inc., discussed in *Life Extension* how "*young-patient specific cells of any kind*" can be used in "*regenerative growth.*" The research hinges on leveraging the capacity of certain cells that can divide indefinitely, which are known as "*immortal reproductive cells*," and preventing those cells from losing that ability.

What makes all of these unbelievable ideas believable is that many of them are building off of concepts that have already been tested.

Many of these treatments and therapies appear far less far-fetched once you consider that they are rooted in science that we are already doing. Cloning is real, of course, and isn't even considered a big deal anymore. Fighting off death is all within our grasp, and progress has been plentiful. We are almost there! And you can thank the incredible amount of cash being thrown at the issue for the progress that has already been made.

As I mentioned earlier, another strategy that is being developed involves using microscopic nanobots to do important biological work in our bloodstreams. The bots used for this kind of work are so small they can fit inside our cells. These *"non-organic"* bots, which just means they are not made out of carbon-based matter, represent some of the most cutting-edge integrations between man and machine. There are many advantages to deploying nanotechnology for biological purposes. Still, perhaps the most important is that these bots are programmable and capable of seamlessly doing so many critical biological functions in tandem with one another.

Let's take an example from *ScienceDirect*, which lays out some pretty remarkable concepts concerning nano-engineering and usage. There, we can see how the lines between organic and inorganic are being blurred more and more every day. *"A surgical nanobot, programmed by a human surgeon, could act as an autonomous on-site surgeon inside the human body. Various functions such as searching for pathology, diagnosis, and removal or correction of [lesions] by nanomanipulation can be performed and coordinated by an on-board computer,"* reads the scientific journal.

Essentially, we are talking about sending in a legion of tiny robots to seek out and destroy, on a molecular level, the things in our body that cause us to age and deteriorate. Even more magnificent is that they can talk to each other and communicate important information in real-time. They can coordinate their attacks like little soldiers taking orders down the chain of command. **It's war, and they are prepared to win**.

Think about the possibilities that this might

have on the medical field. Think about all the things that doctors have struggled to combat over the hundreds of years that modern medicine has existed. Could this irradicate cancer? Could these nanobots correct genetic deformities and imperfections? Could they be used to enhance natural, normal functionality as well? In time, perhaps they can do all of these things. The power these little bots have is truly extraordinary.

## IS AGING EVEN REAL?

*"People don't die of old age, they die of diseases that accompany old age, and they are preventable."*
**Deepak Chopra**

Hear me out on this one. If you look at some of the work and some of the research being done in the field of anti-aging, you will find some pretty amazing things, and one of those things is a new line of thinking that basically rejects the concept of aging altogether. Well, it is more of a rejection of the idea that aging is the reason we *die*, but in either case, the most advanced science has basically shown us that it is impossible to die from "*old age*."

We all die from something, or perhaps several things in conjunction, that ultimately causes our bodily functions to cease. *"Old age"* was just a way for doctors to shorthand, *"We have no idea what really happened because our technology is not there yet, and does it matter, anyway, which of the many, many deteriorating functions truly did this poor sap in?"*

Science is now firmly answering that question with a resounding, *"Yes!"* If we can combat one type of decay, we can probably combat them all. And if we can combat every type of decay and deterioration that takes place in our bodies…well, then what happens? If you ask Aubrey de Grey, perhaps the most brilliant biomedical gerontologist alive and the chief science officer of the SENS Research Foundation, he would tell you that it means immortality—plain and simple.

> **"If changing our world is playing God, it is just one more way in which God made us in His image."**
> **Aubrey de Grey**

Let's talk a little bit about de Grey and his

background before I dive too deeply into his work. You might think he was a descendant of the famed Russian mystic Grigori Rasputin if you saw the man. Now that I think about it, you might think he *is* the famed Russian mystic Grigori Rasputin; the likeness is uncanny, and the line between science and magic has always been pretty blurry, to begin with.

The London-born researcher studied computer science at Cambridge University. From there, he began researching artificial intelligence, notes a biography in *Opalesque*, before moving over to his current fields of study. Although it is probably fair to say that for a guy like de Grey, each field of study he has worked in likely informs the others he is exploring—again, blurred lines abound when we are dealing at such high levels. The difference between biology, chemistry, nanotechnology, and philosophy is more and more indistinguishable by the hour.

Among his many idiosyncrasies, de Grey is in an open marriage and has been reported to be with women both much older and much younger than he is. However, he gives the whole "*age is just a number*" argument a whole new perspective to begin with, so what are a few decades between lovers? He is as rare and unique an individual as you might find anywhere on the planet, and he just might be responsible for the most remarkable scientific breakthrough in the history of humanity.

In March 2021, de Grey took to Twitter to make one of the boldest claims he has made to date. Says the scientist: "***I now think there is a 50% chance that we will reach longevity escape velocity by 2036. After that point (the "Methuselarity"), those who regularly receive the latest rejuvenation therapies will never suffer from age-related ill-health at any age***."

This book was composed in 2021 for those of you keeping score at home.  Those born this year will barely be in high school by 2036.  It is right around the chronological corner.  Think about what might happen if he is right.  He is saying that many of you reading this book right now could potentially *be* one of the *Methuselarity*.  Are you ready for what de Grey is positing?  It begs a lot of questions.

First, would you even choose this *life*style if you could?  How much will it cost you to live forever?  Is it worth it?  How much would you be willing to pay for treatments that would ensure you never die?  Do you want to outlive your loved ones?  Your children?  Should you rip up your will?  The answer to these questions lies at the intersection of science, philosophy, and religion. Just because you can do something, should you?  In this case, yes!

Another exciting thing prospective immortals will need to think about is how they will navigate the new economic realities associated with this new theoretical biological reality. Much of the economy we have built is rooted in the principles of terminal life.  Does the value of something like, for example, a car change if we can roll back aging altogether? Let's hypothesize.

Practically speaking, a car allows people to get from one place to another "*faster*."  Does the value of that benefit decrease as our lives are extended?  What difference does it make if it takes one hour or one day to get from point A to point B if everyone and everything can exist indefinitely?  Stopping or reversing aging will completely reshape the way we view *"time"* since time is relative.  Perhaps we are very far away from dealing with that particular issue, but should we not start thinking in these terms sooner rather than later?  Are gold, diamonds, and Cryptocurrency more valuable than paper money in this new economic reality?  Are they less valuable?  What about the skincare industry?!  There is so much to consider that it can make your head spin.

More specifically, what is de Grey talking about when he makes these bold claims?  For one of the many contributions he has made in this area, de Grey wrote a book called *Ending Aging*, which lays out how he believes science can end this messy business of dying.

*"De Grey's main line of research is into mutations in mitochondrial DNA that cause increased cell stress via production of free radicals. In other words: something that will need to be addressed in a lab rather than in your kitchen or following 'eat healthily and exercise' sort of advice,"* reads the information in *Opalesque*. *"He also elaborates on the*

*essential distinction between preventative/rejuvenating and or curative or palliative treatments: Aging damage will inevitably accumulate, so masking or slowing it, alone, is insufficient to extend life dramatically."*

Essentially, what we are talking about here is not only inhibiting the pathogens that shorten our lives, but actually reversing these effects and rolling back the years we have already aged. In theory, if this practice was honed and perfected, we could choose a state that corresponds to a traditional biological *"age"* and stay at that approximate level forever.

That could be fun. Imagine you are in your early 20s and are still well shy of the brick wall your metabolism will undoubtedly run into in the next decade. You look good, you feel good, and you want to stay this way forever. You can. Of course, it might be fun to see what you look like with that natural salt and pepper hair in your mid-50s, too. See what happens when you get there, and if you don't like it, just roll back the clock and start anew. Or get to somewhere in the middle and see what that looks like on you. Stay there at 35. Or not. You can look and feel however you like! The power would be incredible.

Interestingly, de Grey said that the anti-aging industry's biggest challenges are not born of the science itself, but the financing. Even with the above-stated billionaires pouring in copious amounts of money into the field, de Grey says the problem of funding is still pervasive and operative.

*"It has somewhat alleviated over the past few years, but it's still a really bad problem. Currently, we are still in the mindset as a society of thinking of aging as something very distinct from diseases. We have invented this completely fictitious notion of age-related diseases like Alzheimer's or most cancers and atherosclerosis. So on, as if they were actual diseases that could be cured like infections, when in fact they are simply parts of aging,"* he told *Opalesque.*

In sum, de Grey wants to rewire the way people think about aging and death completely. He wants to put them into different terms and remap the scientific landscape surrounding these ideas. Tall order? Sure. Doable? Absolutely.

## AS EXPANSIVE AS THE UNIVERSE ITSELF

The anti-aging field, as you can see, is quite big, and the strategies being explored span a wide conceptual array. Much of the science deals with doing some very small things in very big ways. Some of these things are cellular-based, like much of what we already touched upon above. **Another cell-based approach, previously discussed and my favorite, is called transdifferentiation, and it has a lot of promise**.

In short, **transdifferentiation-related** therapies, according to Nature.com, involve the conversionary process by which cell types located in one particular organ or tissue can be used in another cell or organ. In these instances, the cells pass over the *"pluripotent cell state*," which can be experimentally induced in addition to happening naturally in certain instances. If induced experimentally, the process could also help combat aging on the cellular level.

Further still, others are exploring using oxygen to manipulate parts of our chromosomes to offset and reverse aging. In Israel, reports *The Resident*, some researchers are using hyperbaric oxygen treatment to lengthen telomeres, which are compounds on the end of chromosomes. According to the report, this process has already had success and could roll back the effects of aging as much as 25 years. A quarter-century younger just by using some high-pressure oxygen! What a time to be alive!

Speaking of rich, eccentric scientists, there are more than a few people who have speculated that Elon Musk has already been experimenting with reversing aging. This, for anyone who has been paying attention to the billionaire space-pioneer, might almost seem like an obvious conclusion based on both his attitude and the evidence.

So, what exactly is going on with Elon Musk? That's a question you are likely to hear a lot. But it behooves us to ask it now, especially considering what we are discussing. An anecdote in *Motor Authority* sums up the existing speculation about the out-of-the-box Tesla CEO.

*"Though filmed nearly 16 years ago, this clip shows a Musk with thinner (nearly male pattern) hair, a mixture of brown and black clothing, and an obsession over a piece of monstrously impressive automotive hardware acquired as a status symbol—all hallmarks of the 55-and-up crowd, hardly the traits of a 27-year-old uber-geek,"* reads the gearhead publication. *" … at age 43, Musk seems much more like the ostensibly 27-year-old self who should have been in the video above. A full head of hair, smooth skin, well-coordinated clothing, and, of course, his upcoming Model 3, a (presumably) attainable and smart-yet-fun sedan for the family of the future."*

See for yourself here what the heck is going on with Musk: if you think about it, Elon has a lot of incentive to try to stop the aging process. If he wants to send someone to Mars, it will be a lot easier to do if they can live forever. It will be a lot easier for *him* to do if he can, himself, live forever.  It's all starting to make sense…build a spaceship, take digital money stored electronically to Mars, and enjoy a nice Earthrise from a Mars mansion made out of gold and diamonds.  Elon Musk, a true futurist, might be ushering in an entirely new chapter of human existence.  After all, if you check out the top of his Twitter feed, you will find a simple yet poignant message about what he wants to do with his company and his work: "*Make humanity a multiplanet species.*"  It appears we might be well on our way.

## THE REALITY OF ARTIFICIAL INTELLIGENCE

*"When you talk to a human in 2035, you'll be talking to someone that's a combination of biological and non-biological intelligence."*
**Ray Kurzweil**

Artificial intelligence used to be little more than fodder for dystopian authors and filmmakers.  It is a massive industry with as much game-changing potential as the work going into reversing aging.  Before we go any further, let's define what artificial intelligence is and consider some of its applications.

Per *Oxford Languages*, provided by Google, artificial intelligence is the "*theory and development of computer systems able to perform tasks that normally require human intelligence, such as visual perception, speech recognition, decision-making, and translation between languages*."

More simply, AI mimics things we normally associate with human behavior. Other related concepts, like machine learning and natural language processing, are more specific applications of artificial intelligence research that deal with data analysis and linguistics. We will talk a little more about those below, as well. Ultimately, the AI space deals with replicating, and in some cases replacing, human beings with inorganic entities. To that end, we are not that far from a future where humans live as long as the imposters we build to replace us.

Economic theorists go back and forth about the impact artificial intelligence and its associated industries will have on the way business is conducted in the future. Will jobs be eliminated?  What will replaced laborers do for income?  Will they be the ones who maintain the AI machines?  Questions like this have led some politicians and policymakers to think long and hard about a *"universal income"* that would protect against seismic shifts in the global economy. (If they were smart, they should start paying it out in Bitcoin now, before it is too late.)

### CAN MACHINES TALK?

Communication is the force that drives the human experience forward.  Some social scientists and theorists believe that communication is the singular defining element of that experience.  Without it, we would be fundamentally different on nearly every level.  Now, much work is being done to elevate the communication abilities of machines to the point that they are indistinguishable from the abilities that human beings have.  Consider this from *Towards Data Science*:

*"Unless you're living under a rock, you'd probably have heard about OpenAI's latest [Generative Pre-trained Transformer]*

*iteration. It has engulfed social media by storm. The reason behind GPT-3's enormous hype right now is due to its mighty model size. Today, it's one of the largest and most powerful machine learning models for natural language processing in the world. Trained on over a trillion words and based on a transformer neural network architecture, the Generative Pre-training model is capable of doing almost any natural language task be it writing prompts, QAs for chatbots or even generating language-specific code."*

A trillion words?! To put it in context, research cited by *Word Counter* indicates average adults use between 20,000 and 35,000 words. Now, we have machines that know multiples upon multiples of the average adult. That is a lot of words to throw around, and you have to wonder how many people will even be able to successfully interact with such an entity.

The implications of having an entity capable of logically organizing thoughts and using that many words are almost impossible for us to conceive. The level of accuracy in communication that is possible in that scenario is staggering. Think about all the different times humans have failed to convey what they were trying to say accurately, and think about all the terrible consequences of those crossed wires. In its apex form, machine learning would virtually eliminate the concept of *"miscommunication."* Be it machines talking to other machines or machines talking to human beings, and they would always say exactly what they mean to say—nothing more and nothing less.

At their peak, these machines should be able to do everything that we can do, and very likely, do it better. So, what does this all mean? Is artificial intelligence going to take over the planet, like in every science fiction movie we have seen in the last few decades? Um... maybe.

In all seriousness, though, AI is being developed to mimic the human brain. This could mean, quite literally, a machine will be able to simulate the entirety of the operations of the human mind. This is either very good news or very bad depending on whom you ask.

# CHAPTER THREE

# LIVING FOREVER MEANS PREPARING FOR THE GREAT RESET

*"He who bets on government and government money bets on 6,000 years of recorded human history."*

*"Thou shall not steal, except for majority vote. It is the politics of two wolves and one sheep voting on what to have for dinner."*
**Both quotes by: Gary North**
**Investment Newsletter Writer**

If the United States government were a private organization, it would be indicted for fraud. Our monetary system is one giant Ponzi scheme. The only thing backing the U.S. Dollar is the fact that the government can tax and confiscate its citizens' income, assets, and resources. However, this house of cards is destined to crumble.

**The government is literally**

*__"creating money out of thin air."__*

The national debt is now over $28 trillion. Gross Domestic Product (GDP) is $21 trillion. GDP is a monetary measure of the market value of all the final goods and services produced in a specific period.

In the year 2000, the U.S. Federal Debt to GDP was 58.46%. Today, as of this writing, that ratio is over 128% and climbing fast. COVID-19 and the global economic meltdown, coupled with huge losses in productivity, have resulted in an alarming amplification of the already troubling debt/GDP ratio.

Another frightening statistic is the increase in the M2 Money Supply since the year 2000. Many of the C-Suite CEOs, let alone the average investor I speak to, have no concept of this shocking statistic that should chill every American to the bone. In economics, the *"money supply"* is the total value of money available in an economy at a point in time. In 2000 the Money Supply was a little over $4.7 trillion, and today it is over $20 trillion and climbing fast! I find this downright horrifying!

The U.S. Government is bringing into existence money (by printing it or creating it digitally) as the need arises. In a recent *60 Minutes* story aired on May 17, 2020, Scott Pelley asked Fed Chairman Jerome Powell:

*"You simply flooded the system with money?"*

**Powell responded, *"Yes, we did. We printed it digitally. As a central bank, we have the ability to create money digitally. And we do that by buying treasury bills or bonds or other government-guaranteed securities, and that actually increases the money supply. We also print actual currency, and we distribute that through the Federal Reserve Bank."***

## THE GOVERNMENT WILL IMPLEMENT RADICAL MEASURES WHEN ITS PONZI-SCHEME FAILS

Currently, the U.S. Government is collecting $3.4 trillion annually in tax revenue. The budget deficit is over $4.5 trillion per year. The government is spending money well over twice as fast as it is collecting it, and it is reasonable to believe that trend will grow exponentially.

*"When the federal government spends more each year than it collects in tax revenues, it has three choices: It can raise taxes, print money, or borrow money. While these actions may benefit politicians, all three options are bad for average Americans."*
**Ron Paul**

*"We could say the government spend like drunken sailors, but that would be unfair to drunken sailors, because the sailors are spending their own money."*
**Ronald Reagan**

Another fact that most Americans are unaware of is the actual national liability, which is a massive multiple of what is reported as the *"national debt."* The actual unfunded national liability is over $162 trillion, including $21 trillion in Social Security liability and $34 trillion in Medicare liability. If you add up the total assets of all American citizens, the total comes to $161 trillion. Our country has a negative net worth, which over time is going to grow and grow. Every man, woman, and child—even a newborn baby—owes $500,000 as our debt stands today.

The current U.S. Dollar will eventually have to be **RESET**.

Confiscation of your assets is also on the horizon, especially if you consider the exponentially increasing $162 trillion national liability. The Dollar's collapse is inevitable. The Government will simply **RESET** everything. **Your money in the bank will disappear**. Your property will be seized. If you are lucky, you will still be able to remain in your house. However, it's conceivable that the government may order you to take in the homeless, even if your home is not a large one.

Does this sound wacky? Maybe . . .

But recall that in 1933, U.S. Citizens were required to relinquish their gold bullion for ***"government promissory notes,"*** or in plain language U.S. Currency. Executive Order 6102, signed by President Roosevelt, required all persons to deliver to the government on or before May 1, 1933, all but a small amount of their privately owned gold coins, gold bullion, and gold certificates to the Federal Reserve.

**Failure to comply was punishable by ten years in prison**. This was **NOT** an act of Congress...it was an order by the President of the United States acting under the equivalent of martial law.

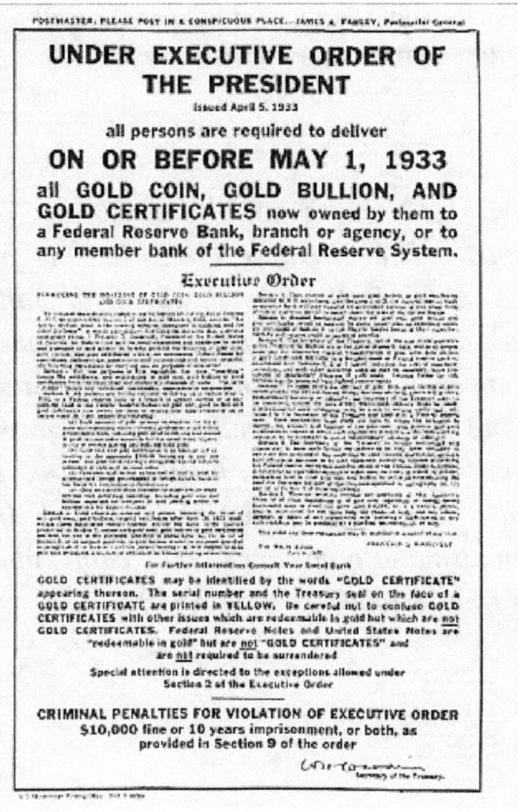

POSTMASTER: PLEASE POST IN A CONSPICUOUS PLACE. JAMES A. FARLEY, Postmaster General

# UNDER EXECUTIVE ORDER OF THE PRESIDENT

Issued April 5, 1933

all persons are required to deliver

# ON OR BEFORE MAY 1, 1933

**all GOLD COIN, GOLD BULLION, AND GOLD CERTIFICATES** now owned by them to a Federal Reserve Bank, branch or agency, or to any member bank of the Federal Reserve System.

### Executive Order

For Further Information Consult Your Local Bank

GOLD CERTIFICATES may be identified by the words "GOLD CERTIFICATE" appearing thereon. The serial number and the Treasury seal on the face of a GOLD CERTIFICATE are printed in YELLOW. Be careful not to confuse GOLD CERTIFICATES with other issues which are redeemable in gold but which are not GOLD CERTIFICATES. Federal Reserve Notes and United States Notes are "redeemable in gold" but are not "GOLD CERTIFICATES" and are not required to be surrendered

Special attention is directed to the exceptions allowed under Section 2 of the Executive Order

## CRIMINAL PENALTIES FOR VIOLATION OF EXECUTIVE ORDER

$10,000 fine or 10 years imprisonment, or both, as provided in Section 9 of the order

Secretary of the Treasury.

Deemed by the Press "*The Great Robbery of 1933,*" the only exception to this involuntary forfeiture was that citizens were allowed to keep gold coins for the purpose of maintaining a rare coin collection (more about this later in this book).

*"Sometimes people don't want to hear the truth because they don't want their illusions destroyed."*
**Friedrich Nietzsche**

**SHARK TALK**: *The Great Reset* **is inevitable. The Greatest Ponzi-Scheme of all—the U.S. Dollar, is destined to fail. Granted, it may take ten years or more, but it will happen. It may be unnerving and horrifying to face the reality of this grave situation, but to survive in the future, a prudent individual should invest in semi-numismatic gold coins, rare coins, and e-coins (the "money" of the future).**

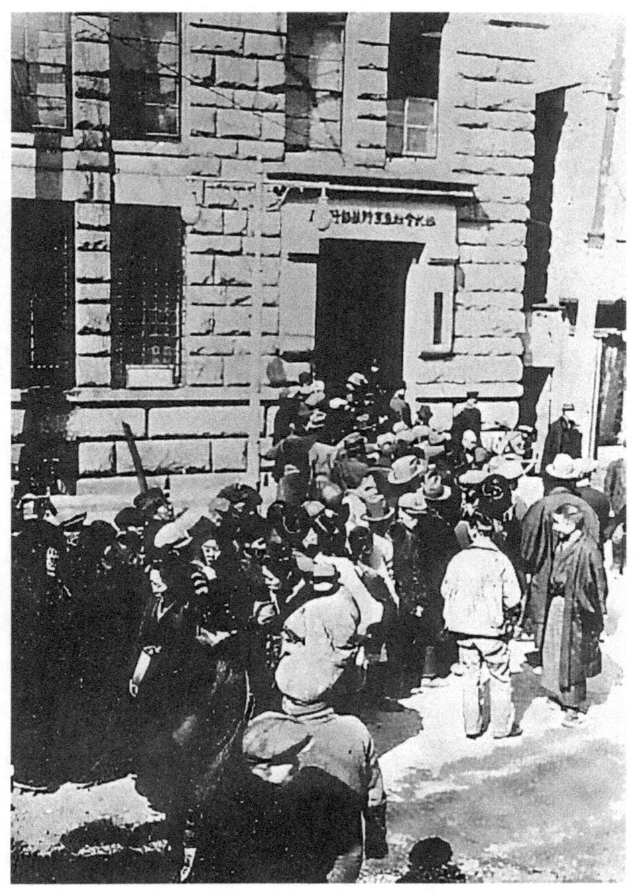

To prepare for THE GREAT RESET in the long-term and to profit substantially **RIGHT NOW**, you need to think and invest as a billionaire would. I recommend investing no less than 25% of your liquid net-worth into semi-numismatic gold coins. Another 10% to 25% of your assets should be allocated to high-performing numismatic rarities. Finally, another 15% to 20% should be utilized for hedging with Cryptocurrency. In the upcoming chapters, I will discuss each category specifically.

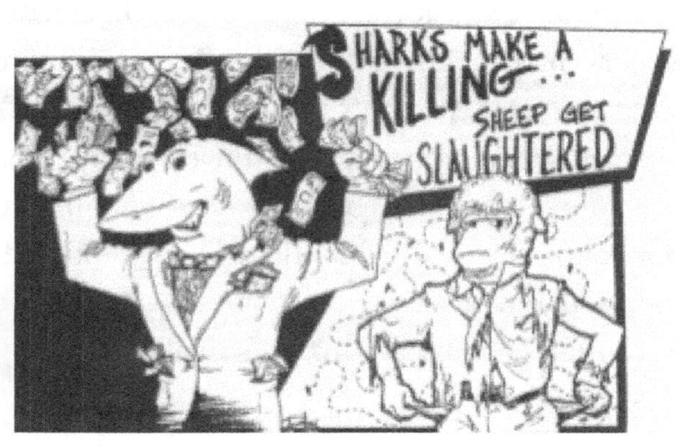


*"Mankind invented the atomic bomb, but no mouse would ever construct a mousetrap."*
**Albert Einstein**

*"It (Corona Virus) has been used by certain forces, inimical to families and to the freedom of states, to advance their evil agenda. These forces tell us that we are now the subjects of the so-called 'Great Reset,' the 'New Normal'."*
**Cardinal Raymond Burke**

During fifty years from 300 AD to about 350 AD, the price of gold compared to the Roman Denari rose 42,000%!   Like the U.S. government is doing today, Rome *"printed money"* to pay for various government-subsidized programs. Of course, history had taught us that the Roman Empire eventually fell when its currency was RESET. History seems to be repeating itself today. The U.S. government is bound to extinction, but our currency will fail first. Any prudent individual will realize THE GREAT RESET is coming and prepare for its arrival.

## SKEPTICAL?
## MORE LESSONS FROM OUR HISTORICAL PAST  AS HISTORY REPEATS ITSELF OVER AND OVER AGAIN

In the early 1700s, the country of France was in tremendous debt. Like the United States today, the interest payments owed greatly exceeded taxes collected. Duke d'Orleans, the de facto ruler at that time, conspired with a consummate con-man named John Law to *"create money out of thin air."* Sound familiar?

Law, a womanizer, degenerate gambler, and sociopathic murderer who happened to be a fugitive from justice, launched his sinister scheme. The Duke, desperate to save France's economy, allowed Law to create his own bank. *Banque Générale,* as it was called, was permitted, under the color of French law, to print and create its own currency.

At first, Law's bank and its currency were very successful. Law was hailed as the *"Warren Buffet"* of his time. He was considered a financial prodigy. Everything he touched turned to gold. He quickly became one of the richest men in the entire free world.

The conspiracy continued; under the express authority (and personal request) of the Duke, Law's bank diluted the nation's currency supply. Using nothing more than a printing press, Law created more and more of the nation's fiat currency. As this Ponzi scheme continued, France seemed to prosper and grow financially. The world viewed France as a haven of financial stability.

Like Alexander the Great, the Roman Empire (and the U.S. government today), France was spending and spending with little restraint. But things looked good. Construction was everywhere. The people were happy.

Then it happened: hyperinflation caused the cost of consumer goods to rise thousands of percentage points. The wealthy and elite,

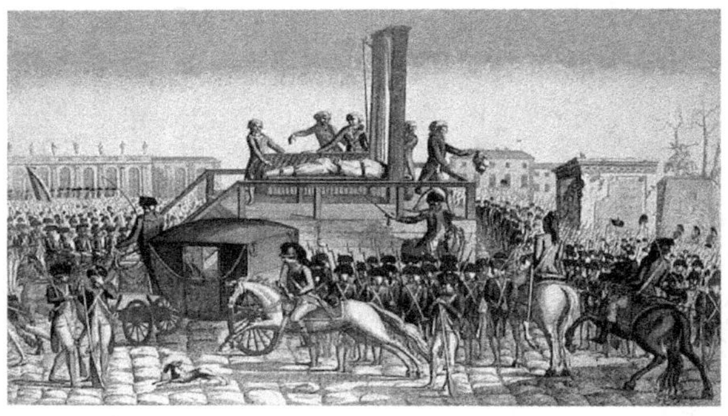

sensing the collapse of French paper currency, started redeeming their worthless fiat currency for gold. **In 1720, just as Roosevelt did in 1933, the French government arbitrarily made it illegal to own gold**. France enacted its GREAT RESET. Gold, silver, diamonds, and almost all commodities of value were required to be forfeited to the government. If you did not comply, well...the French had the guillotine.

France and most of Europe plunged into economic chaos. John Law became the *"Bernie Madoff"* of his time.

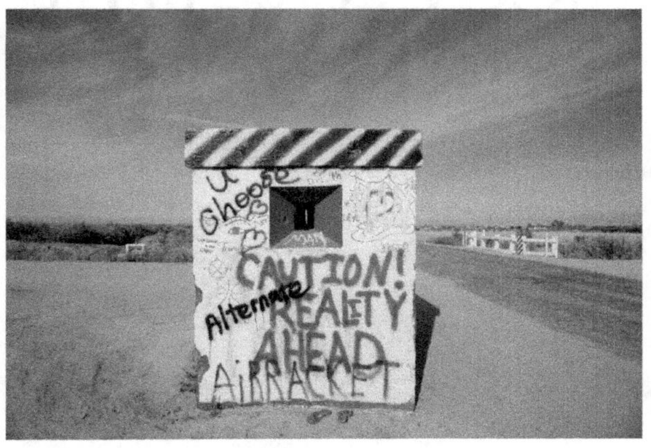

# CHAPTER FOUR

# YOUR PLAN TO THRIVE & LIVE FOREVER

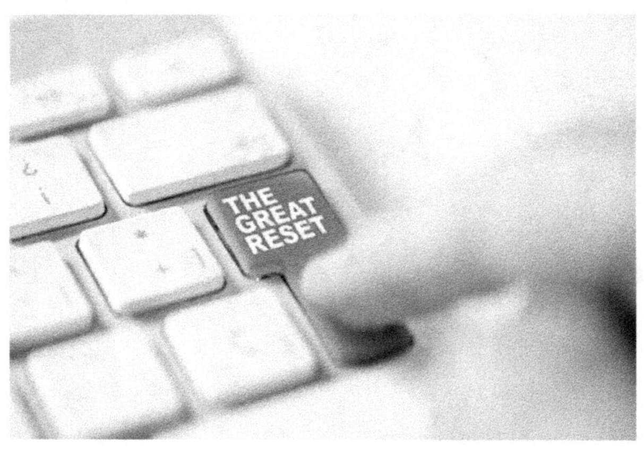


*"Intelligence is the ability to adapt to change."*
**Stephen Hawking**

*"Change is the only constant in life. One's ability to adapt to those changes will determine your*

The world is changing at an incredibly rapid pace. If you are going to Thrive During the Great Reset you must **adapt**. The coming global currency reset is a topic that is not talked about much, if at all, in the mainstream media.

I believe that during President Biden's administration, we will experience **Phase 1** of The Great Reset—exorbitant increases in taxes, skyrocketing energy costs, and food prices shooting through the roof. The Federal Reserve will create more and more fiat currency. Tens of trillions of dollars will be *"created out of thin air"* to pay for social welfare programs, pay sovereign debts, and to fund failing businesses.

The national debt will grow exponentially. Many banks, insurance companies,and innumerable cities and state governments will go into bankruptcy.

It should be obvious, *"unless you are blind and walking around without a cane,"* that the current monetary system will eventually collapse. We are headed towards a socialist dictatorship. The government is able to increase the money supply at will, and the masses will suffer because of it.

**A Shark, however, not only adapts and survives, but a Shark will prosper**. I see The Great Reset as an opportunity—an unprecedented opportunity to obtain great wealth and prosperity.

## PHASE 1
## THE NEXT FOUR YEARS

*"Everything government touches turns to crap."*
**Ringo Starr**

During the next four years, I expect the buying power of the U.S. Dollar to deteriorate. Wages will go up, and there will be more government handouts, but ultimately the masses will have to settle for less. There will be food shortages and power blackouts in some geographical regions. Inflation will erode your capital.

Our military will suffer major cutbacks (a foolish move to save money). As our military weakens, enemies of our republic will become emboldened and test the mettle of our government to see how America will react/respond.  Our ally, Israel, will be shunned (BIG MISTAKE), and the United States will get in bed with certain rogue nations in the Middle East to avoid possible conflicts while insipidly attempting to appease the nations that represent socialism/Communism.  The above is just the tip of the proverbial iceberg.  I haven't even addressed unconstitutional legislation or radical regulations.


There will be extreme, inclement weather conditions (an increase of earthquakes, tornados, hurricanes, floods, wildfires, droughts, etc.), which will be due to "*global warming*" or "*climate change.*"  The radical right's insistence that climate change is a myth is outrageous and dangerous.  Follow the science.

There will also be a lack of quality healthcare. Conservatives and anyone who thinks the wrong way will find themselves routinely being persecuted, castigated, and admonished. There will be inequitable anger leveled towards them and their carefree lifestyles. With regard to the elderly, Social Security increases will be stifled, and there will be mega-inflation to cope with. Myriad farms and businesses will fail, not to mention the horrendous physical, mental, emotional toll caused by intolerable strife, stress, and duress that will face the average American. Firearms will be confiscated from law-abiding citizens, as has happened in EVERY historical case whenever totalitarian governments have been formulated. Additionally, First Amendment rights will be drastically stifled, more so than ever before in our lifetime.

What do I base my dire predictions upon? Historically, EVERY nation, kingdom, republic, state, city, or township that has followed these exact same ideologies has ultimately ended up collapsing in an undignified heap. Ancient Rome, for example, had a population of over a million people. For an ancient city, that was remarkable. The innovations and technologies developed by the Roman Empire were state-of-the-art for the times. The world was in awe. It was the greatest civilization the world had ever seen. The Romans were a world power for centuries. But the Roman Emperors started debasing their currency, and Rome collapsed—the population of Rome was eventually reduced to around eight thousand people. The very wealthy made a getaway to safe-havens, but most perished. The lesson that history taught us is not being heeded. Man is repeating his mistakes over and over again up until this very day.

Remember my story about the Zimbabwe monetary crisis? Well, Steve Hanke, a member of the *Cato Institute*, estimated the accumulated inflation rate as of November 14, 2008, at 89.7 quintillion percent. Between October 24 and November 14, prices in Zimbabwe increased 170-200 fold each week. And even more recently was the rapid destruction of Venezuela. Get ready for a long and bumpy ride. A similar scenario will materialize, which the majority of our populace will never believe or comprehend could ever happen here in our beloved United States. You might SAVE this missive for posterity.

The central bank's continuation of "*creating*" money is a crime against humanity. It is a losing proposition. The U.S. Dollar and the Federal Reserve are destined to fail. It is essential to open your eyes and understand that, given the current conditions, the value of the money that we earn and keep will be Reset—it is only a matter of time. The collapse of the U.S. dollar and all world currencies is getting closer and closer. **Remember the tulip**.

Gita Gopinath, Director of the *International Monetary Fund's* Department of Studies, described the current economy as *"... the worst global contraction in peacetime since the Great Depression. Due to the partial nature of the rebound, more than 150 economies are expected to have per capita incomes below their 2019-2021 levels."* The IMF official adds *"... that the projected accumulated production loss during 2020-2025 in relation to the levels forecast before the pandemic continues to be substantial."*

Governments of the world, especially the United States, are bankrupting their country. They are destroying their currency without actually caring for the long-term economic health of their population. A bankrupt government cannot provide national security. The government's efforts are focused on holding onto power. They do this by increasing the money supply with no regard to long-term consequences. However, we are heading towards the end game. **Central banks are a cancer. Their horrific practices are unconscionable. The fate of the American dollar looks daunting.**

## PHASE 2
## THE EROSION OF CIVIL LIBERTIES

*"It is easy to believe in freedom of speech for those*
*with whom we agree."*
**Leo McKern**

The second phase of The Great Reset will be the start of a surge of inflation never before seen in the United States. In the 1970s and 1980s, double-digit inflation plagued the nation. Those numbers will seem agreeable in the future, as triple and quadruple-digit inflation threatens our currency.

The U.S. dollar has continued to be created with no backing, to the point of no return. In Phase 2, the central banks that print money *"out of thin air"* will become dinosaurs. As the population ages, social security and medicare obligations will become unaffordable. The elderly without income or assets will suffer tremendously. The sick and infirm will be left to die, as there will be no money for healthcare for those without assets.

No one will trust government-issued money. Blockchain will eliminate the SWIFT system that regulates international bank transfers. The exponential debt growth will become totally unsustainable and unpayable. All major currencies of the world will fail. The world's stock markets will plummet. Economic activity will decline rapidly. Gold, tangible assets, and Cryptocurrency will explode in value! The only non-tangible asset that will retain any value is cryptocurrency; it is the tulip that keeps blooming.

Political sacrificial lambs will be ripe for slaughter.    You will be told how to think. Honest, peaceful debate and opposition to the "*norm*" will be considered "*radical thinking.*" After years of lies and deception, government leaders will resort to drastic and violent methods to keep power.    Civil liberties, freedom of the press, and free speech will become subject to the control of radical groups. Free will—well, enjoy it while it lasts.    Even today, circa 2021, most Americans are willing to sacrifice civil liberties in the name of what they think is "*right*" or facilitating "*their way of thinking*"...**as long as they are the civil liberties of someone else!!!**


## PHASE 3
## THE BIOTECH REVOLUTION

*"Government cripples you, then hands*
*you a crutch and says,*
*'See, if it wasn't for us, you couldn't walk.'"*
**Harry Browne**

The technological and biological revolution will take hold. In this final phase, the government will be able to literally read your mind. The Neural Link will scan your brain for *"wrong thinking."* AI will dominate every facet of your life. The *"Singularity"* will arrive, but most of the world will have no idea about the wonderful advancements made in biotechnology and nanotechnology. The rich/poor divide will be ever-increasing. These economic inequalities between the classes will unleash violent riots with increasing frequency and intensity. Through government intervention to quell the masses, wealth distribution will incorporate profound and radical reforms. The government will confiscate assets. The very wealthy, however, will maintain their power and financial status.

Sharks will survive. Sharks have been with us for 450 million and will be the last creatures on Planet Earth to live. Sharks adapt.

The plan is simple. If you want to Thrive During The Great Reset, you need to adapt and change with the times. You need to be a Shark!


## YOUR PLAN
### Adapt—Make Drastic and Immediate Changes

*"The weak fall, but the strong will remain and never go under."*
**Anne Frank**


## <u>STRATEGY ONE</u>—Accumulate gold.

Economic disaster will be a reality. Each passing day brings us closer to global monetary collapse.

You will see a worldwide depression in the near future, and gold will be one of the few fungible forms of money. I wholeheartedly recommend gold, but I don't recommend TRADING. I recommend that you buy semi-numismatic gold coins as an insurance policy against disaster.  Accumulate gold to protect your family, as Federal Reserve Notes and other world currencies will eventually lose all their value. **Banks cannot print gold.** An old Chinese proverb says *"Real gold is not afraid of the melting pot."*

Gold will protect the purchasing power of your portfolio. Gold is a succinct form of wealth.  A world government can not simply create it *"out of thin air."*  Gold does not accrue gargantuan indebtedness   or   unfunded   government liabilities.   Gold  does  not  care  about  the speeches or promises of politicians.  Gold has a sustained  and  unparalleled  track  record  at preserving wealth.

Physical gold is money.  Don't buy gold to speculate  on  it,  or  to  wait  for  substantial appreciation and then sell.  Buy gold to hold in preparation for The Great Reset. One day you will be able to exchange your semi-numismatic gold coins for food, medical care, or whatever else is needed.

## <u>STRATEGY TWO</u>—Accumulate a collection of rare coins and art.

Individuals that control America's wealth adore art and collectibles. Rare coins offer enormous attractions, including being beautiful pieces of art offering historical significance, and in certain cases, spectacular investment potential. Coins have one major advantage—they are portable and easy to transport and trade, compared to a rare *Picasso* or another valuable piece of art. One day you may need to trade your rarity to get medicine or food for your children. Perhaps your desirable rare coin or spectacular piece of art might be traded for something incredibly valuable, like nanobots placed in your body when the *"Singularity"* arrives.

*"Collecting numismatic items causes one to better appreciate such diverse disciplines as history, geography, mathematics, and fiscal and artistic considerations. As a bonus, items collected*

## <u>STRATEGY THREE</u>—Buy Crypto Currency.

Buy Bitcoin and VOGEL coin. When currency is devalued and/or totally collapses, Cryptocurrency will be the new form of *"money."* The government can print money. Bitcoin can be mined, but there is a limit of 21 million units. And, remember currently, 19 million Bitcoin have already been mined, leaving only a tiny amount left to dilute the market.



## <u>STRATEGY FOUR</u>—Make staying in perfect health a priority in life.

You can't enjoy wealth if you're not in good

health. If you want to make it to the "*Singularity,*" I will repeat what I said earlier in this book: be a health nut! Physical fitness and exercise are the most important keys to a healthy body. It is also the basis of superior and creative intellectual achievement.

Personally, I eat five to ten raw vegetables every day and three to five pieces of fruit. I eat egg whites and if I eat bread, it has to be whole wheat. I refuse to eat any carbohydrate that is not complex, and I almost always avoid any product made with sugar. In addition, I exercise vigorously six day per week. I can't afford to die. It would wreck my image.

*"The only way to keep your health is to eat what you don't want, drink what you don't like, and do what you'd rather not."*
**Mark Twain**

*"When I first started out, I was considered a crackpot. The doctors used to say, 'Don't go to that Jack LaLanne, you'll get hemorrhoids, you won't get an erection, you women will look like men, you athletes will get muscle-bound'—this is what I had to go through."*
**Jack LaLanne**

# STRATEGY FIVE—Make lots of friends.

Friends bring more happiness into our lives and have a huge impact on our mental health. Good friends relieve stress. They prevent loneliness and isolation. Developing close friendships will have a powerful impact on your physical health.

Each new friendship you make opens up new doors and opportunities. Every new friend you meet can teach you something you didn't know. Learn from them.

Every new friend you make becomes a possibility that you will be inducted into the *"Singularity."*

*"Do I not destroy my enemies when I make them my friends?"*

**Abraham Lincoln**

**SHARK TALK**—The Reset of the U.S. Dollar will benefit those who hold tangible assets and Cryptocurrencies! The coming decade promises a very profitable market for gold, collectibles, and Cryptocurrency. Stay healthy if you want to make the "*Singularity.*" Make as many friends as possible. Continue to educate yourself every day. Pray and enjoy life.

> *"It is not the strongest or the most intelligent who will survive, but those who can best manage change."*
> Leon C. Megginson

# CHAPTER FIVE

# Becoming a Shark

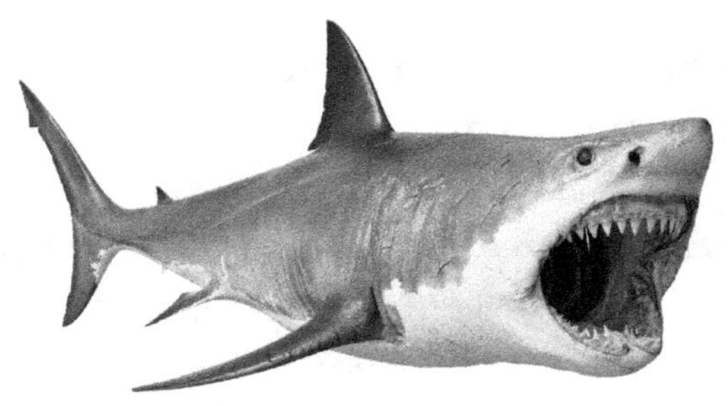

All of this leads up to my big finale. The climax of everything we have discussed so far in this book. When all the chips are down, we are talking about survival—both biological and economical. One thing I know for sure: **Sharks** survive. Again, they have been here for 450 million years.

When you think of the ferocious underwater creature that is all but universally revered, known as the **Shark,** what are the first few things that come to mind? Fierce, very likely.

Predatory, perhaps? Feared. Loved. Savage. All of these are perfectly reasonable ways to describe the biological entity known as a Shark. Well, I posit this: you can be a Shark, too. Yup, that's right, even a human being can be a Shark.

In my terms, a Shark is someone like sports owner, outspoken television personality, and billionaire-genius investor Mark Cuban. Cuban is such a Shark he is literally on a television show called *Shark Tank*. Cuban is smart, savvy, and creative—the holy trinity of Sharkdom. People like Mark Cuban do not wait for opportunities to fall into their lap; they seek them out. They hunt them. Human Sharks are just as predatory as their seafaring counterparts, except they have way nicer houses and drive much nicer cars.

One thing that sets a Shark apart from everything else is its uncanny instinct to survive. Moreover, in the face of adversity, they not only survive but thrive. Do you think something like a little-old nuclear blast is going to stop a Shark? Think again. The economic collapse of the world economy—no problem.

Political unrest? Social fissuring? It doesn't matter; these bad boys know how to ADAPT! There is a reason they have been living on this planet for 450 million years. They are a genetic marvel. You can be that, too.

One of the things I am trying to accomplish here is to teach you how to be a **Shark,** and be just as successful as the famous ones you've heard about. And I know what I am talking about, so listen up.

Long before ABC put *Shark Tank* in the living rooms of American families, I was talking about surviving the real-world version of it in my second book, which was themed, illustrated, and about, you guessed it, financial **Sharks.** That was in 1994, in case you are keeping score at home. I have been enamored with the concept for a long time, and with good reason. It makes perfect sense in the context of both finance and biology.

My upcoming podcast, **Shark TV®**, is already being produced as we speak. There I will thoroughly explain, from top to bottom, how to survive and thrive as an investment hunter.

There I am going to layout in full measure what it takes to win in the game of finance.  It is not going to be easy, but each and every one of you can do it with the proper hunger and instinct for blood in the water.

**Sharks** are proficient at a lot of things. **Sharks** know how to invest their money in sectors that are going to GROW. **Sharks** know what to avoid.  They know a scam, a hoax, or a con before anyone else. They know what not to do as well as they know what they must do to succeed.  They know the difference between being "*rich*" and creating wealth.  They know how to build a future.  They know how to create generational success that can withstand the harsh realities of global politics, economic recessions, environmental disasters, and whatever the universe throws at them. **Remember, a Shark ALWAYS survives**.

Another element of being a **Shark** that has gone largely unexplored is how a **Shark** takes care of their body.  A true **Shark** survives not only because they have the financial means to do so, but because they have the mind, the body, and the spirit to endure.  I want you to be wealthy, but I also want you to be healthy. We talked a lot about anti-aging in this book, and we even talked about how to reverse the whole thing altogether. If you are truly going to thrive as a **Shark**, you are going to need to stay abreast of all the developments in this fantastic, emerging space.

If you want to learn more about how to do this, I highly suggest you sign up for **Shark Talk®**, my e-zine. There, you will be treated to updates on the key topics we touched upon in this book: finance and trade, artificial intelligence, strategies to reverse aging, money-making, health, wealth, and The Great Reset. These topics are the pulse of our new reality. If you can master these, you can put yourself in a position to overcome anything the coming centuries have to throw at you.

One final note on Mark Cuban, whom I admire greatly. He is a wildly successful individual and deserves all the credit in the world, but he does *not* get to take credit for the **Shark** analogy that has driven much of my earlier work. I am not saying I invented using the

**Shark** to symbolize being financially slick, sharp, and intelligent, but I did.

All kidding aside, I do want you all to succeed. The world is constantly changing. One minute we are trading potatoes for goats; the next minute, it is a piece of paper with a dead person's picture on it, and someday soon, it will be neither of the above. How will you know what to do? How will you know what is right? Information, instinct, and absolute devotion to better yourself and evolve every day. You have it within you to do this; all that is left is to put into practice everything we talked about. You got this! You are going to be great!

Finally, I will leave you **Sharks** with a little story to close out all we have talked about in this book. **The Great Reset** is coming, and I want you all to be ready for it, just like I was … ever since I was nine years old.

## WHAT THE GREAT RESET MEANS FOR YOU

As we wind down the book, I want you to think about everything you have read so far. Now ask yourself this: "*What does The Great Reset mean to me?*"  Is it going to be an economic crisis?  Is it going to be an environmental disaster?  Will it be science-born? Religious? Will it be all of the above?

For me, it comes down to a simple reality: the current economic model is shifting rapidly away from fiat currency towards digital money. This conflict will pit nations against one another.  It will force institutions, banks, regulators, lobbyists, businesses, and even regular people to fight for economic survival. **Adapt or die**.  For many people, things are going to get harder before they get easier. Not everyone is well-positioned to take part in this fight.  One side will lose, and when they do, they will lose badly.  Don't be on the wrong side of history.  You must be prepared for the seismic shifts on the horizon.

The good news is that you will be on the *right* side of history. You are a **Shark** now.  Let me leave you with a cheeky little story about when I first realized I was a **Shark**.  (In honor of the fact, of course, that you just right now realized that YOU are a **Shark**).

The year was 1969. I was all but nine years old sitting in Mrs. Powsner's class, and she was trying to explain *"Russian"* authoritarian-communism to a bunch of elementary school kids. Spoiler alert: she was not doing a good job of it. She said that if we were in Russia right then, we would all be poor, have no luxury items, and have nothing of any real value to our names. I told her (remember, I'm nine years old here) that she had absolutely, positively no idea what she was talking about. I told my teacher, to her face, that she didn't know anything. It was wild. But sadly, it was true! I told her, *"You ignorant slut! Get your facts straight! You are babbling about the Soviet Union, not Russia. And I am a **Shark**, and one day the owner of the Dallas Mavericks is going to make a television show about me!"* OK, I might have stretched out that last part, but you get the idea.

What I really told Mrs. Powsner was that I am creative, I am smart, and I know how to survive and adapt. I communicated how myopically she was thinking. If I were in the communist Soviet Union, I said, ***"I would be***

*the Minister of Propaganda and be plenty
wealthy and rich.*" Why? Because I'm a
**Shark**, and I want you to all become **Sharks**
with me. So let's get to it! Biden's
administration—no problem. Reset—no
problem. A **Shark** will adapt. A **Shark** will
prosper.

The good news is **Sharks** will be able to
transdifferentiate by 2045. **Sharks** will avail
themselves of the only viable solution to
aging—nanotechnology!

**Sharks will cheat death**

# A **Shark** is a Singulatarian!

*"A Singulatarian is one who understands the
Singularity and who has reflected on its
implications for his or her own life."*
**Ray Kurzweil**

I coined the term nano-cellular regeneration in
2021, but I believe it will be a household word
in ten years. This is exciting news! By 2045,
we'll be in the midst of a technical revolution
the likes of which humanity has never seen.

A **Shark** is a *"Singulatarian."*  As a **Shark,** you will be alive long after ALL fiat money has come and gone. Because you are aware of nano-cellular regeneration and the coming *"Singularity,"* you will be prepared to take advantage of everything this marvelous era of science offers.

If you're under 65 and in good health, there is every reason to believe that immortality can be yours in two short decades!  If you're a **Shark,** you've already got a friend in me.  Soon you will be able to tune in to **Shark TV®**.  I will announce when the first episode will be on YouTube in my newsletter: **Shark Talk®**...be sure to get a free e-subscription; details are in the Appendix.   I'll keep you up to date on all the latest developments involving your wallet and your future as an immortal.   We'll definitely have a few laughs along the way. I am always a lot of fun!   Always smart, scientific, real, and entertaining.  I want you to be a loyal fan!

In this book, we've talked about THE GREAT RESET, and about how to prepare yourself for it by hoarding gold.  You learned that paper money is backed by nothing and will inevitably fail as governments abuse it.  But now you're ready to move beyond such flimsy and insecure fiat money and buy things of tangible value. You've read the book; you're ready to start diversifying!

I also explained why collectible coins are a great way to diversify.  They have both intrinsic value (as precious metal) and emotional value (as objects coveted by collectors).  With this guide, you have all you need to get started...start collecting precious coins, artwork, etc.! You will have a blast! Remember—a Real Man owns a Faberge Egg.  Contact me today, and I will hook you up.  If you want to buy or sell gold or any precious collectible, you should consider having this **Shark**  (me) represent your best interest.

As we approach the "*Singularity*," technology will continue to become more and more integrated into our lives. It's only natural that a digital currency would arise.  If Bitcoin is not part of your portfolio, there's every reason to consider it.  The future is now, but you are ready for it!

By 2045, the world will have changed in unprecedented ways.  But only those who are wealthy and connected will be able to take advantage of the greatest scientific advances of all time—the chance of everlasting life.  Elon Musk will be there, and Mark Cuban, and Peter Thiel.  Will you?

As **SHARKS**, you're prepared for the "*Singularity*."  And that means an unbelievable opportunity that will be available to you if you don't let anything stand in your way if you filter out the lies, and if you just reach out and grab it!  You will be healthy, wealthy, surrounded by friends, and eager for your coming immortality!

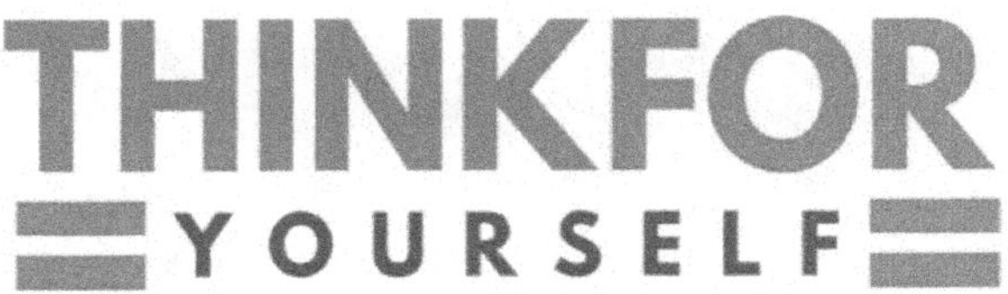

# APPENDIX

## SHARK TALK®

I publish a newsletter called **SHARK TALK®**. All readers of this book are invited to send for a FREE subscription to my highly acclaimed e-zine which will be sent directly to your email address.  Learn about what is really going on in American finance  and the latest technological advancements as we move forward to **THE GREAT RESET** and The "*Singularity*" on an up-to-the-minute basis.

If you read my book,  you will receive a FREE subscription just for asking.

### To subscribe,  please visit:

**https://sharktv.tv/talk**

# SHARK TV®

Do YOU want to learn how to masterfully navigate the deep waters of high-finance, technology, health and more? Then you are DEFINITELY going to want to check out my soon-to-be released podcast: **SHARK TV®**. Point-blank, there is NOTHING you are going to find anywhere that is quite like it.

On **SHARK TV®**, my brand-new podcast, you will learn how to turn ideas into actions, turn money into wealth and turn yourself from just another fish into a fearsome sea-predator. With **SHARK TV®**, you will learn how to BECOME a **Shark**. The world is changing; everything we thought we know about how it works, from the very atoms that create us, to the BIG ideas that drive commerce, business, politics and policy, is being turned on its head. Changes are coming, and if you can't swim fast enough to keep up, you're going to get eaten!

I will teach how to avoid the fish traps, scams, scoundrels and anyone else trying to bait you and take you for a ride. **SHARK TV®** is aimed squarely at giving you the tools you will need to survive in a savage space. If you want success in this life, you are going to have to learn how to do what it takes to beat the odds, beat the competition and even BEAT THE OTHER SHARKS!

No topic is off limits on this game-changing podcast—we are going to talk about everything from Cryptocurrency to diamonds, gold, silver, The Great Reset, artificial intelligence, anti-aging, anti-matter, wealth, health, medicine, magic, mayhem and so much more. If it matters, we got it covered top to bottom. Our guests are atop their fields, our news is breaking, and our content is as fresh as the finest chum money can buy. You CANNOT afford to miss what we have coming if you want to win in the ocean!

Also, be sure to sign up for my e-zine, which is going to cover all of those above e-mentioned hot topics and more. Stay up to date on how to stay healthy and fit, learn about cutting-edge anti-aging treatments that are literally changing the way we view science, and keep up to date on all the news coming out of Wall Street, Main Street the Moon, Mars and more! Tech updates? Check. Science news? Check. Learning how to create real, actual, generational wealth? Check, Check and Check!

And the best part, **SHARK TALK®** is as free as the ocean is vast. What a deal! That means if you live forever—and we ALL know that is coming—signing up today is nothing short of a trillion dollar value! Who doesn't want a trillion dollar value? Right?!

If YOU want to stay in the know and give yourself a fair chance in the deep-blue arena, you are going to NEED **SHARK TV®** *and* **SHARK TALK®**. These two incredible offerings are going to change your life! If you know what's good for you, you will get swimming right now by clicking the links below. For all you fish out there, time is wasting. Get to it!!!

**SharkTV®** will be premiering on YouTube in the near future. For up-to-date information announcing  the date of the premier episode, subscribe to **SharkTalk®**

## To subscribe, please visit:

<u>https://sharktv.tv/talk</u>

# NOTES AND QUESTIONS
# FOR MR. VOGEL:


Please do not hesitate to write or call me if you need help buying or selling gold, rare coins, artwork, or any other collectible. I can be reached at 802-546-1133. Or you can email me at david@sharktv.tv.  Send snail mail to Shark TV®, Box 736, Wolfeboro, NH 03896

# About the Author

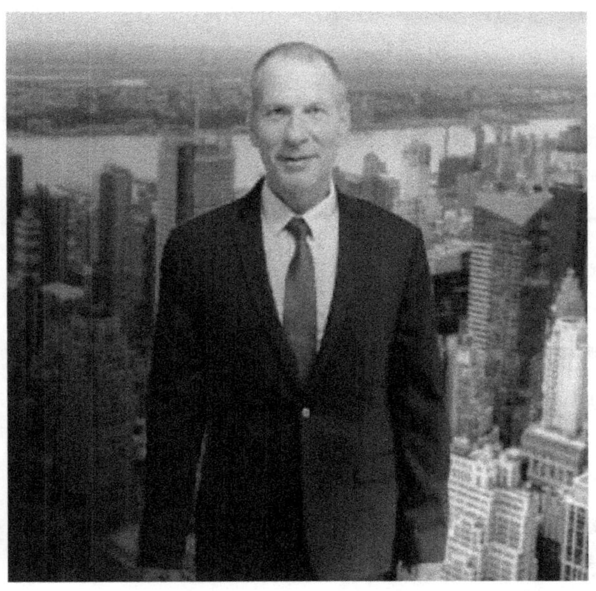

David A. Vogel was born in 1960 and has been involved in the finance, bullion, rare coin, and art business since the age of 14. Recently, he started an Artificial Intelligence marketing company, and his AI is used by some of the largest corporations in the world.

David started his career by founding a lucrative mail-order business in the mid to late 1970s. In 1986, he joined Heritage Rare Coin

Galleries and quickly became their number one senior numismatist. In late 1988, David left Heritage to form his own firm. During his career, he has had the privilege of serving countless satisfied customers and has personally handled sales of some of the finest and rarest coins extant.

David's strategies effectively place him among the world's most prudent expert professional numismatists. In addition to being one of our nation's foremost authorities on buying and selling rare coins, gold, and art, he has recently taken an interest in one of the newest forms of money—Bitcoin, electronic money, and non-fungible tokens (NFT's). David, well-versed in all financial markets, marketing, and business administration, is an author, lecturer, and consultant.

In addition, David publishes newsletters analyzing economic and political trends, which he believes are essential in making a prudent decision concerning any financial market. David is also a technology buff and studies quantum physics and nanotechnology. He is an outspoken consumer advocate and a member of many political, religious, and charitable organizations.

David lives in Alton, New Hampshire, and has five grown children. Besides family activities, David's other interests include weightlifting, aerobics, and collecting art. David's greatest love (besides his family) is swimming in ice-cold waters.

**Email David at david@sharktv.tv or call him at 802-546-1133.**

www.ingramcontent.com/pod-product-compliance
Lightning Source LLC
Chambersburg PA
CBHW060634080726
47818CB00004B/138